Study Guide and
Computerized Learning Resource
to Accompany

NURSING RESEARCH
Methods, Critical Appraisal, and Utilization

Study Guide and Computerized Learning Resource to Accompany

NURSING RESEARCH
Methods, Critical Appraisal, and Utilization

Kathleen Rose-Grippa, PhD, RN
Professor and Director
School of Nursing
Ohio University
Athens, Ohio

Mary Jo Gorney-Moreno, PhD, RN
Professor
School of Nursing
San Jose State University
San Jose, California

Computerized Learning Resource by

Mary Jo Gorney-Moreno, PhD, RN

FOURTH EDITION

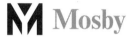

St. Louis Baltimore Boston Carlsbad Chicago Naples New York Philadelphia Portland
London Madrid Mexico City Singapore Sydney Tokyo Toronto Wiesbaden

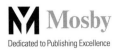

Mosby
Dedicated to Publishing Excellence

A Times Mirror
Company

Publisher: Nancy L. Coon
Editor: Loren S. Wilson
Developmental Editor: Aimee E. Loewe
Project Manager: Gayle Morris
Designer: Yael Kats
Manufacturing Manager: Linda Ierardi

FOURTH EDITION

Printed in the United States of America
Composition by Wordbench

Mosby–Year Book, Inc.
11830 Westline Industrial Drive
St. Louis, Missouri 63146

International Standard Book Number 0-8151-2810-X

Book Code 31130

98 99 00 01 02 / 9 8 7 6 5 4 3 2 1

Contributors

Sharon A. Denham, DSN, RN
Associate Professor
School of Nursing
Ohio University
Athens, Ohio

Joy Edwards-Beckett, PhD, DNSc, RN
Independent Research Consultant
Westerville, Ohio

Ann Marttinen Doordan, PhD, CRRN
Professor, Advanced Placement Coordinator
School of Nursing
San Jose State University
San Jose, California

Mary Jo Gorney-Moreno, PhD, RN
Professor
School of Nursing
San Jose State University
San Jose, California

Sharon S. Mullen, PhD, RN
Assistant Professor
School of Nursing
Ohio University
Athens, Ohio

Martha Rock, PhD, RN
Assistant Professor
School of Nursing
Ohio University
Athens, Ohio

Kathleen Rose-Grippa, PhD, RN
Professor and Director
School of Nursing
Ohio University
Athens, Ohio

DEDICATION

To Paul, who picks up the pieces when I can't.
To Michael, Matthew, Sarah, Lydia, Caitlin, Gregory, Ric, Carolyn, and Rebekah whose
   questions keep me stimulated and whose lives keep me organizationally nimble.
To Mary Jo goes a special thanks—she knows why.
To Loren and Aimee—thank you, thank you, thank you!

Kathleen Rose-Grippa

I want to take this opportunity to thank my students in Nursing Research 128 at San Jose State University, especially those in the Television Education classes, for their excitement, enthusiasm, and interest in research and for always "pushing the envelope," helping me learn how to coordinate E-mail systems and download files. It has been a journey that we have shared through many phone calls and E-mails when the files didn't transfer smoothly.

I want to thank my husband, Manuel, and daughter, Elizabeth, without whose unwavering support this edition, especially the CD-ROM, would not be completed. Thanks also to John and Maggie Ybarra for providing excellent writing facilities in their home. A special thanks to Victor Moreno, Artist/Designer, Wild Card Art Works, Federal Way, Washington for creating the icons.

Thanks to San Jose State University, which has truly become "The Metropolitan University of Silicon Valley" under the leadership of President Robert Caret; whose training and support through Morning Shu at the Alquist Center and Dr. Baird at the Institute of Teaching and Learning have given me the information and motivation to actively participate in the technology and information revolution. Thanks to my School Director, Dr. Bobbye Gorenberg, for a stable assignment. Having the opportunity to repeatedly teach the Undergraduate Nursing Research Course has given me insight into student learning patterns and problems on this topic.

Finally, thanks to Loren Wilson at Mosby whose incisive answers clarified questions, and Aimee Loewe for her patience, persistence, and diligence.

Mary Jo Gorney-Moreno

Contents

Also included . . .

CD-ROM by Mary Jo Gorney-Moreno

Introduction

Change, change, change seems to be the byword as we enter the next millennium in health care and communications. In keeping with this spirit, we have made changes in this edition:

1. We added icons (graphics) so you can quickly key into special topics. The Icon Gallery on p. xi provides a key to determining each icon's function.

2. More international examples are provided. We really enjoy having a large international audience and have included examples from Sweden, the United Kingdom, and Australia.

3. Our inclusion of references and exercises for websites may encourage you to look at clinical research through a wide angle lens. There is considerable work occurring and websites provide us with very current resources.

4. We have included a free CD-ROM that you can use on an IBM/Pentium or Macintosh/Apple computer. It contains activities that supplement those in the study guide.

5. The WWW home pages that appear in the appendix are also new.

What an incredible time to be a nurse! For the first time the focus of clinicians, researchers, and accrediting agencies is directed toward outcomes. All partners in the health care industry recognize that we need a better understanding of the link between interventions and outcomes. If "what we do matters," then outcome studies can only become more important to practice.

The link between interventions and outcomes, combined with the knowledge explosion, has created a new world, which is opening its doors to you. Never before in health care has there been a knowledge explosion of this magnitude. In the not too distant past it was accepted that without on-going study, a professional's knowledge would become outdated in 5 years. Now, 2 years is the currently accepted time limit, and the prediction is that by the year 2005 knowledge will be outdated in 12 hours. We have 7 years to develop the skills to access and use just-in-time knowledge. A critical understanding of all readily available information will be even more essential than it is today. This study guide will lead you in the beginning stages of developing such a critical understanding.

The activities in this book and the accompanying CD-ROM are designed to assist you in evaluating the research you read so that you are prepared to undertake the critical analysis of studies. As you practice the critiquing skills addressed in this study guide, you will be strengthening your ability to make practice-based decisions grounded in nursing theory and research.

General Directions

1. Complete each chapter and the activities in that chapter sequentially. This *Study Guide* is designed so that you build on the knowledge gained in Chapter 1 to complete the activities in Chapter 2, and so forth. The activities are designed to give you the opportunity to apply the knowledge learned in the textbook and actually use this knowledge to solve problems, thereby gaining increased confidence that comes only from working through each chapter.

2. Follow the specific directions that precede each activity. Be certain that you have the resources needed to complete the activity before you begin that activity.

3. Do the posttest after all of the chapter's activities have been completed. If in doubt, check with your instructor for the answers. If you answer 85% of the questions correctly, you can feel very confident that you have grasped the essential material presented in the chapter.

4. Clarify any questions, confusion, or concerns you may have with your instructor, or write or E-mail the authors of this *Study Guide*.

5. We recommend that you read the textbook chapter first, then complete the *Study Guide* activities for that chapter, and finally complete the supplemental activities on the CD-ROM. (*Note:* The activities on the CD-ROM are different from those found in this *Study Guide*.)

The Activity Answers Are in the Back of This Book

Answers in a workbook such as this are not "cut and dry" like answers in a math book. Many times you are asked to make a judgment call about a particular problem. If your judgment differs from that of the authors, review the criteria that you used to make your decision. Determine if you followed a logical progression of steps to reach your conclusion. If not, rework the activity. If the process you followed appears logical, and your answer remains different, remember that even experts may disagree on many of the judgment calls in nursing research. There will continue to be many "gray areas." If you average an 85% agreement with the authors, you can be sure that you are on the right track and should feel very confident about your level of expertise.

Mary Jo Gorney-Moreno, PhD, RN
E-mail: Gorney@SJSUVM1.SJSU.EDU
Kathleen Rose-Grippa, PhD, RN
E-mail: grippa@oak.cats.ohiou.edu

Icon Gallery

In an effort to attract your attention to a special point, the following icons have been included in this *Study Guide*. These icons will alert you to special ideas, suggestions, or circumstances that may not seem obvious. They will help you discover clues from seasoned research critiquers.

 Critical Thinking—An activity that requires you to use reasoning to make a decision, or analyze, or synthesize the information that you have read in the text and apply this thinking to a case study or situation in the *Study Guide*.

 Critiquing Criteria—A point is being illustrated by demonstrating the utilization of critiquing criteria found in the textbook.

 Hot Tip—Insider information or suggestions that may assist you in completing an activity.

 Qualitative—This activity or example is appropriate only to qualitative research designs.

 Quantitative—This activity or example is appropriate only to quantitative research designs.

 Technology Resource—This activity involves knowledge of computer technology or Internet resources.

 World Wide Web Resource—Either an Internet address or an example from an Internet source is supplied.

The Role of Research in Nursing

1

Mary Jo Gorney-Moreno

Introduction

One goal of this chapter in the study guide is to assist you in reviewing the material presented in Chapter 1 of the text written by LoBiondo-Wood and Haber. A second and more fundamental goal is to provide you with an opportunity to begin practicing the role of a critical consumer of research. Succeeding chapters in this workbook fine-tune your ability to evaluate research studies critically.

Learning Outcomes

On completion of this chapter, the student should be able to do the following:
- Utilize research terminology appropriately.
- Identify the research roles associated with each of the educational preparation levels of nurses.
- Identify significant events in the history of nursing research.
- Identify nursing's role in future trends in research.
- Critically analyze the significance of nursing research to own nursing role.

Activity 1

Match the term in Column B with the appropriate phrase in Column A. Each term will only be used once.
This may be a good time to review the glossary.

Column A

1. _____ Systematic inquiry into possible relationships among particular phenomena

2. _____ One who reads critically and applies research findings in nursing practice

3. _____ Examines the effects of nursing care on patient outcomes in a systematic process

4. _____ Critically evaluates a research report's content based on a set of criteria to evaluate the scientific merit for application

5. _____ Implementation of a scientifically sound research-based innovation into clinical practice

6. _____ Theoretical or pure research that generates tests and expands theories that explain phenomena

Column B

a. Critique

b. Consumer

c. Research

d. Clinical

e. Basic research

f. Research utilization

Check your answers with those in Appendix A, Chapter 1.

Activity 2

Listed below are specific research activities. Using the American Nurses' Association (ANA) guidelines, indicate which group of nurses has the primary responsibility for each activity. Use the abbreviations from the key provided.

Key: A = Associate degree   C = Master's degree
         B = Baccalaureate degree   D = Doctoral degree

1. _____ Design and conduct research studies.

2. _____ Identify nursing problems needing investigation.

3. _____ Assist others in applying nursing's scientific knowledge.

4. _____ Develop methods of scientific inquiry.

5. _____ Assist in data collection activities.

6. _____ Be a knowledgeable consumer of research.

7. _____ Demonstrate an awareness of value of nursing research.

8. _____ Collaborate with an experienced researcher in proposal development, data analysis, and interpretation.

9. _____ Promote the integration of research into clinical practice.

Check your answers with those in Appendix A, Chapter 1.

Activity 3

1. Examine the four articles that are in the appendices of the LoBiondo-Wood and Haber book. What is the educational preparation of the person(s) responsible for each study? List the degrees (i.e., RN, BSN, MS, PhD, or DNSc) of each author next to the author's name. Remember, this information is usually found in the short biographical paragraph on the first page or at the end of the article.

   a. Wikblad, _____ and Anderson, _____

   b. Draucker, _____ and Petrovic, _____

   c. Rudy, _____; Daly, _____; Douglas, _____; Montenegro, _____;

      Song, _____; and Dyer _____

   d. Ward, _____ and Misiewicz, _____

2. In what way does this information regarding the educational preparation of the researcher influence your thinking about the study? Before drawing any conclusions, answer the following questions:

   a. Is the first author's education preparation at the doctoral level? (Circle the correct answer.)

      Appendix A   Yes or No

      Appendix B   Yes or No

Appendix C   Yes or No

Appendix D   Yes or No

The general assumption is that the first author carries the major responsibility for the research.

b.   If there are other authors is there other evidence of his or her role in the research (such as data collector) and is this congruent with ANA's prescription for roles based on educational preparation?

Appendix A

Appendix B

Appendix C

Appendix D

c. Were any of the studies funded by external funding agencies? Write below which study and agency provided external funding, if any. This would indicate that the research proposal had been reviewed by an external source and deemed meritorious enough to receive funding to complete the study.

Appendix A

Appendix B

Appendix C

Appendix D

Check your answers with those in Appendix A, Chapter 1.

Activity 4

Complete the following crossword puzzle as you would any other crossword puzzle. Note that if more than one word is needed in an answer, there will be no blank spaces between the two (or more) words of the name or phrase. Refer to the text for help.

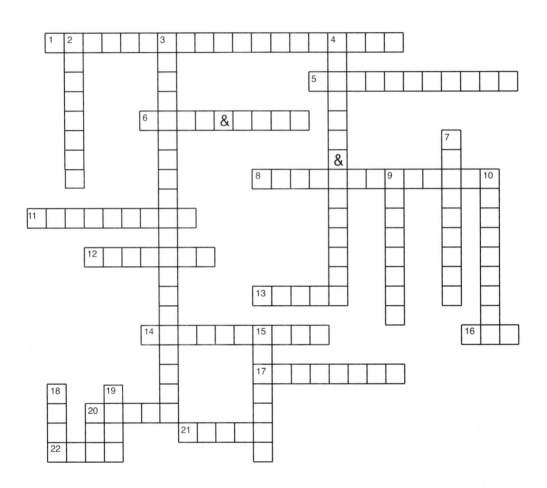

Across

1. Collected and analyzed data on the health status of the British Army during the Crimean War.
5. The 1920s saw much of this type of research published in the *American Journal of Nursing (AJN)*. (2 words)
6. The research of _____ and _____ led to New York City's hiring of school nurses. (*Note:* Use ampersand [&] between names.)
8. In 1981 the ANA published guidelines for the role of the nurse in research. What synonym for the word research was used in the title? (*Hint:* Check reference list).
11. One of the first topics of clinically oriented research in the early half of the century.
12. Researcher who conducted a classic clinically oriented study of safety and cost savings of early hospital discharge of very-low-birth-weight infants.
13. A decade of increased emphasis on practice-oriented research. (*Numerical*)
14. Lydia Hall's research led to the creation of this totally nurse-run health care facility.
16. This organization sponsored the first Nursing Research Conference in 1967. (*Initials only*)
17. Lamb (1992) reports that a series of _____ studies demonstrated that the community-based nursing care delivery model has a positive impact on quality outcomes.
20. Earliest nursing research course taught in this decade. (*Numerical*)
21. Historically this group has been excluded from clinical research and is likely to be a major funding source in the future.
22. *Healthy People* _____ published by the Public Health Service. (*Numerical*)

Down

2. _____ Report, published in 1970, concluded that more practice-oriented and education-oriented research was necessary.
3. Focus of US Public Health funded nursing research in the 1950s. (*Abbreviate last plural word*)
4. They studied aspects of thanatology, the care of dying patients, and their caretakers. (*Note:* Use ampersand [&] between names.)
7. First nurse to keep systematic written records of patient care (such records are critical to retrospective research). (*First initial and last name*)
9. _____ report in 1923 sponsored by Rockefeller Foundation emphasized the need for nursing education to move into the university.
10. Focus of nursing research between 1900 and 1950.
15. National Center for _____ Research established in 1986 at NIH.
18. Year *Clinical Practice Guidelines: Urinary Incontinence, Acute Pain Management, and Pressure Ulcers published by AHCPR. (Numerical)*
19. First year of the decade in which the journal of *Nursing Research* was first published. (*Numerical*)
20. Currently there are more than _____ research centers in 32 states. (*Numerical*)

Check your answers with those in Appendix A, Chapter 1.

 AHCPR's guidelines are available at their World Wide Web site (i.e., http://www.ahcpr.gov//) or by phone at 1-800-358-9295; from outside the United States call (410) 381-3150. (See Appendix B for the home page.)

Activity 5

The Department of Health and Human Services published *Healthy People 2000* in 1992. The report is a compilation of 22 expert working groups who specified as one objective: "to reduce physical abuse directed at women by male partners to no more than 27 per 1,000 couple." One example of the way nursing is helping to achieve this objective is through studies and publications such as the 1993 *Nursing Research* article, "Physical and emotional abuse in pregnancy: a comparison of adult and teen-age women" by Parker. Other ways nursing and nurse researchers are helping to address this objective are:

a.

b.

c.

d.

Check your answers with those in Appendix A, Chapter 1.

Activity 6

Now that you have read the chapter, answer the following questions in your own words in a way that is meaningful to you. As usual the workbook authors will share their answers with you in the back of this text.

1. Why is knowing about nursing research important to me as practicing nurse?

2. How could I use the information gained from the Brooten (1986) study in my clinical practice?

3. How will nurses produce depth in nursing science?

4. If you were asked to give testimony about your practice to the local city council, state assembly, or senate what research information would you like to have to assist you in presenting the testimony?

Posttest

1. Listed below are descriptions of research activities being carried out by nurses. Indicate in the space in front of each description for which of the following the action is most appropriate:
A = An associate degree prepared nurse
B = A baccalaureate degree prepared nurse
C = A master's prepared nurse
D = A doctorally prepared nurse

a. _____ Provide expert consulting to a unit that is considering changing the unit's practice on the care of decubitus ulcers based on the results from a series of studies.

b. _____ Take and record the blood pressures of hypertensive clients during their monthly visits to the clinic. Blood pressures are taken as part of a study on the effects of contingency contracting by a nurse researcher.

c. _____ To understand and critically appraise research studies to discriminate whether a study is provocative or whether the findings have sufficient support to be considered for utilization.

d. _____ Design and conduct research studies to expand nursing knowledge such as the Anderson (1993) study, *The Parenting Profile Assessment: Screening for Child Abuse.*

2. Match the terms in Column B with the appropriate phrase in Column A. Not all terms from Column B will be used.

Column A

1. _____ First nursing doctoral program began at Teacher's College, Columbia University

2. _____ National Institute for Nursing Research authorized

3. _____ Nightingale studied mortality rates of British in Crimean War

4. _____ NINR areas of special interest for these years include testing community-based nursing models

5. _____ *Nursing Research* publication began

Column B

A. 1995 to 1999

B. Mid and Late 19th century

C. 1992

D. 1920 to 1929

E. 1993

F. 1952

G. 1900

H. 2000

The answers to the posttest are in the *Instructor's Resource Manual*.
Please check with your instructor for these answers.

References

Anderson C: The parenting profile assessment: screening for child abuse, *Appl Nurs Res* 6(1):31-38, 1993.

Draucker B, Petrovic K: Healing of adult male survivors of childhood sexual abuse, *Image: J Nurs Schol* 28:325-330, 1996.

Parker B et al: Physical and emotional abuse in pregnancy: a comparison of adult and teen-age women, *Nurs Res* 42(3):173-178, 1993.

Rudy EB et al: Patient outcomes for the chronically critically ill: special care unit versus intensive care unit, *Nurs Res* 44:324-331, 1995.

US Department of Health and Human Services: *Healthy people 2000: summary report*, No. PH591-50213, Boston, 1992, Jones & Bartlett.

Ward SE, Berry PE, Misiewicz H: Concerns about analgesics among patients and family caregivers in a hospice setting, *Res Nurs Health* 19:205-211, 1996.

Wikblad K, Anderson B: A comparison of three wound dressings in patients undergoing heart surgery, *Nurs Res* 44:312-316, 1995.

Overview of the Research Process

2

Mary Jo Gorney-Moreno

Introduction

Tools are needed for whatever task one sets out to do. Sometimes the tools are relatively simple and concrete (e.g., a pencil). Other times the tools are abstract and more difficult to describe. The tools you need to critically consider research fit into the abstract tool category. They are tools of the mind (e.g., critical thinking and critical reading tools). The following activities are designed to help you recognize and use these tools.

Learning Outcomes

On completion of this chapter, the student should be able to do the following:
* Identify the characteristics of critical thinking.
* Identify the components of critical reading.
* Use the components of critical thinking and reading on selected passages.
* Identify the format and style of quantitative versus qualitative research articles.

Activity 1

Complete each item with the appropriate word or phrase from the text.

1. Critical thinking is a(n) _____ (rational; irrational) process.

2. A noted theorist, Paul (1995) states that critical thinking is a(n) _____ (active; passive), intellectually engaging process in which the reader participates in an _____ (inner; outer) dialogue with the writer.

3. To read critically, readers must enter the point of view of someone other than themselves and instead must enter _____.

4. Nursing students are first introduced to critical thinking skills through utilization of the _____ process of assessment, diagnosis, planning, intervention, and evaluation.

5. What is the minimum number of readings of a research article recommended in the text?

_____

Check your answers with those in Appendix A, Chapter 2.

Activity 2

Match the term in column B with the appropriate phrase in Column A. Terms from Column B will be used more than once.

Column A   **Column B**

1. _____ To get a general sense of the material   a. Critical thinking (CT)

2. _____ Clarify unfamiliar terms with text   b. Critical reading (CR)

3. _____ Using constructive skepticism

4. _____ Question assumptions

5. _____ Rational examination of ideas

6. _____ Thinking about your own thinking

Check your answers with those in Appendix A, Chapter 2.

Activity 3

1. The process of critical reading has four levels, or stages, of understanding. The levels are listed below in a scrambled order. Rearrange the components into the correct order.

   Scrambled order:
   Synthesis Understanding
   Preliminary Understanding
   Comprehensive Understanding
   Analysis Understanding

   Appropriate order:

   a. _____

   b. _____

   c. _____

   d. _____

2. Synthesis Understanding, or putting it all together, is one of the final steps in critical reading. It can easily be broken into a series of activities that work best if completed in order. The steps are listed below in a scrambled order; rearrange each set into the appropriate order.

   Scrambled order:
   Staple the summary to the top of copied article
   Summarize study in own words
   Complete one handwritten 5 x 8 card per study
   Review your notes on the copy
   Read the article for the fourth time

   Appropriate order:

   a. _____

   b. _____

   c. _____

   d. _____

   e. _____

Check your answers with those in Appendix A, Chapter 2.

Activity 4

Determine whether the article in Appendix D (Ward SE, Berry PE, and Misiewicz, 1996) is a quantitative or qualitative study. Utilize the following points to determine if the study you are reading is of a quantitative design. First answer *yes* or *no* for each item, then summarize your thoughts in a paragraph.

1. Hypotheses are stated or implied in the article.   Yes   No

2. The terms *control* and *treatment* group appear.   Yes   No

3. The terms *survey*, *correlational*, or *ex post facto* are used. (*Note:* Read the glossary definitions for help in answering this question.)   Yes   No

4. The term *random* or *convenience* is mentioned in relation to the sample.   Yes   No

5. Variables are measured by instruments or tools.   Yes   No

6. Reliability and validity of instruments are discussed.   Yes   No

7. Statistical analyses are used.   Yes   No

   Summary

Check your answers with those in Appendix A, Chapter 2.

Activity 5

You are reading the Rudy et al (1995) article in Appendix C and find a reference to the sociotechnical theory: "To replicate these results it is necessary to recognize the sociotechnical theory that underpins the SCU environment of care (Daly et al, 1991; Happ, 1993). . . ." You have never heard about this theory before, but believe that you could understand the article better if you could learn about it. How will you quickly find out about this theory?

Check your answers with those in Appendix A, Chapter 2.

Posttest

1. In analyzing research articles it is important to remember that the researcher may _____ (omit; vary) the steps slightly, but that the steps must still be systematically addressed.

2. To critically read a research study, the reader must have skilled reading, writing, and reasoning abilities. Use these abilities to read the following abstract, then identify concepts, clarify any unfamiliar concepts or terms, and question any assumptions or rationale presented.

   This article describes risky drug and sexual behavior and mental health characteristics in a sample of 240 homeless or drug-recovering women and their most immediate sources of social support. . . . Fifty-one percent of the women and 31% of their support sources had Center for Epidemiological Studies Depression Scale (CES-D) scores of 27 or greater, suggesting a high level of depressive disorders in both samples. Similarly, 76% of the women and 59% of their support sources had psychological well-being scores below a standard clinical cutoff point. These data suggest that homeless and impoverished women turn to individuals who are themselves at high risk for emotional distress and risky behaviors as their main sources of support. (Nyamathi A, Flaskerud J, and Leake B, 1997)

   a. Identify concepts.

   b. List any unfamiliar concepts or terms that you would need to clarify.

   c. What assumptions or rationale would you question?

3. Quantitative and qualitative articles will vary a great deal in format and style when they appear in journals. The following statements will focus your attention on these differences and help you to distinguish between the two major types of research. Answer the following questions by inserting the correct term from the list provided. Not all terms will be used.

Used
Generate hypotheses
Statistical tests
Conducted
Test a hypothesis
Analyze themes or concepts

a. The primary difference between the two is that the qualitative study does not
_____ but may _____.

b. An additional major difference is in the way the literature reviews are
_____ and _____ in the
study.

The answers to the posttest are in the *Instructor's Resource Manual*.
Please check with your instructor for these answers.

References

Daly BJ et al: Development of a special care unit for chronically critically ill patients, *Heart Lung* 20:45-51, 1991.

Happ MB: Sociotechnical systems theory: analysis and application for nursing administration, *J Nurs Admin* 23:54, 1993.

Nyamathi A, Flaskerud J, Leake B: HIV-Risk behaviors and mental health characteristics among homeless or drug-recovering women and their closest sources of social support, *Nurs Res* 46:133-137, 1997.

Paul RW: *Critical thinking: how to prepare students for a rapidly changing world*, Santa Rosa, CA, 1995, Foundation of Critical Thinking.

Rudy EB et al: Patient outcomes for the chronically critically ill: special care unit versus intensive care unit, *Nurs Res* 44:324-331, 1995.

Ward SE, Berry PE, Misiewicz H: Concerns about analgesics among patients and family caregivers in a hospice setting, *Res Nurs Health* 19:205-211, 1996.

Research Problems and Hypotheses

3

Mary Jo Gorney-Moreno

Introduction

This chapter focuses on the problem statement and hypothesis. If done correctly, a problem statement can be very helpful to you as a consumer of nursing research because it very concisely (usually in one or two sentences) describes the essence of the research study. For the nurse who considers using the results of a given study in practice, the two primary concerns are to locate the problem statement and critique that problem statement. The hypothesis or the research questions provide the most succinct link between the underlying theoretical base and the research design. Thus, its analysis is pivotal to the analysis of the entire research study.

Learning Outcomes

On completion of this chapter, the student should be able to do the following:
- Identify terms related to the problem statement and hypothesis.
- Compare and contrast the characteristics of research problems and hypotheses.
- Differentiate between a "good" problem statement and a problem statement with limitations.
- Distinguish between each of the following:
  a. Research hypothesis
  b. Statistical hypothesis
  c. Research question
  d. Directional hypothesis
  e. Nondirectional hypothesis
- Distinguish between independent and dependent variables.
- Apply critiquing criteria to the evaluation of a problem statement in a research report.

Activity 1

Match the terms in Column B to the appropriate phrase in Column A. Not all terms from column B will be used.

Column A

1. _____ An interrogative sentence or declarative statement about the relationship between two or more variables

2. _____ The variable that has the presumed effect on the second variable

3. _____ The variable that is not manipulated

4. _____ A property of the problem that indicates it is measurable by either qualitative or quantitative methods

5. _____ The concepts or properties that are operationalized and studied

Column B

a. Testability

b. Independent variable

c. Variables

d. Dependent variable

e. Problem statement

f. Hypothesis

Check your answers with those in Appendix A, Chapter 3.

Activity 2

A good problem statement exhibits four characteristics. Read the problem statements below and examine them to determine if each of the four criteria is present. Following each problem statement is a list representing the four criteria (a-d). Circle *yes* or *no* to indicate whether each criterion is met.

The problem statement:
a. Clearly and unambiguously identifies the variables under consideration
b. Clearly expresses the variables' relationship to each other
c. Specifies the nature of the population being studied
d. Implies the possibility of empirical testing

1. The purpose of this study was to describe the association between the marital relationship and the health of the wife with chronic fatigue and immune dysfunction syndrome (CFIDS) (Goodwin, 1997).
   Criterion a: Yes No
   Criterion b: Yes No
   Criterion c: Yes No
   Criterion d: Yes No

2. This study examined the effects of an individualized computerized testing system for baccalaureate nursing students enrolled in health assessment and obstetrics-women's health during a 3-year period (Bloom and Trice, 1997).
Criterion a: Yes   No
Criterion b: Yes   No
Criterion c: Yes   No
Criterion d: Yes   No

3. This study was an examination of perceptions about the causes of coronary artery disease and the timeline of the disease among 105 patients hospitalized because of myocardial infarction or for coronary angiography and receiving the diagnosis of coronary artery disease (Zerwic JJ, King KB, and Wiasowicz GS, 1997).
Criterion a: Yes   No
Criterion b: Yes   No
Criterion c: Yes   No
Criterion d: Yes   No

Check your answers with those in Appendix A, Chapter 3.

Activity 3

The ability to distinguish between independent and dependent variables is a crucial preliminary step to determine whether a research hypothesis is a succinct statement of the relationship between two variables. Identify the variables in the following examples. Decide which is the independent (presumed cause) variable and which is the dependent (presumed effect) variable.

1. The use of cathode ray terminals (CRTs) increases the incidence of birth defects.

   a.   Independent variable:

   b.   Dependent variable:

2. Individuals with birth defects have a higher incidence of independence-dependence conflicts than individuals without birth defects.

   a.   Independent variable:

   b.   Dependent variable:

3. What is the relationship between daily moderate consumption of white wine and serum cholesterol levels?

   a.   Independent variable:

   b.   Dependent variable:

4. Problem-oriented recording leads to more effective patient care than narrative recording.

   a.   Independent variable:

   b.   Dependent variable:

5. Nurses and physicians differ in the way they view the extended-role concept for nurses.

   a.   Independent variable:

   b.   Dependent variable:

6. The purpose of this study was to determine the extent to which sex, age, height, and weight predict selected physiologic outcomes, namely, forced expiratory volume in one second (FEV1), hemoglobin concentration, food intake, serum glucose concentration, total serum cholesterol concentration, and cancer-related weight change (Brown, Knapp, and Radke, 1997).

   a.   Independent variables:

   b.   Dependent variables:

Check your answers with those in Appendix A, Chapter 3.

Activity 4

Now take each hypothesis (or research question) from Activity 3 and label it with the appropriate abbreviation from the key provided. More than one abbreviation from the key may be used to describe each item.

Key: RQ = Research question
        RP = Research problem
        DH = Directional hypothesis
        NDH = Nondirectional hypothesis
        Hr = Research hypothesis
        Ho = Statistical hypothesis

1. _____   The use of cathode ray terminals (CRTs) increases the incidence of birth defects.

2. _____   Individuals with birth defects have a higher incidence of independence-dependence conflicts than individuals without birth defects.

3. _____   What is the relationship between daily moderate consumption of white wine and serum cholesterol levels?

4. _____ Problem-oriented recording leads to more effective patient care than narrative recording.

5. _____ Nurses and physicians differ in the way they view the extended-role concept for nurses.

6. _____ The purpose of this study was to determine the extent to which sex, age, height, and weight predict selected physiologic outcomes, namely, forced expiratory volume in one second (FEV1), hemoglobin concentration, food intake, serum glucose concentration, total serum cholesterol concentration, and cancer-related weight change (Brown, Knapp, and Radke, 1997).

Check your answers with those in Appendix A, Chapter 3.

Activity 5

The next step is to practice writing hypotheses of different types. Return to the first three of the six hypotheses/questions/problems you labeled in Activity 4. Each was labeled as a specific type of hypothesis, research question, or problem statement. Rewrite each of the first three to meet the conditions of the remaining four types of questions or hypotheses. The first problem is partially completed to provide an example.

Problem 1: The use of cathode ray terminals (CRTs) increases the incidence of birth defects.

DH   The use of CRTs increases the incidence of birth defects.

NDH   The use of CRTs influences the incidence of birth defects.

Hr   The use of CRTs increases the incidence of birth defects.

RQ

Ho

Problem 2: Individuals with birth defects have a higher incidence of independence-dependence conflicts than individuals without birth defects.

DH

NDH

Hr

RQ

Ho

Problem 3: What is the relationship between daily moderate consumption of white wine and serum cholesterol levels?

DH

NDH

Hr

RQ

Ho

Check your answers with those in Appendix A, Chapter 3.

Activity 6

Critique the following hypotheses. There were two hypotheses tested in this study.

1. *Hypothesis I:* There will be significant improvement in the dressing independence of cognitively impaired nursing home residents following implementation of strategies to promote independence in dressing (SPID) (Beck et al, 1997).

    a. Is the hypothesis clearly stated in a declarative form?
        Yes No
    b. Are the independent and dependent variables identified in the statement of the hypothesis?
        Yes No
    c. Are the variables measurable or potentially measurable?
        Yes No

d.   Is the hypothesis stated in such a way that it is testable?
Yes No

e.   Is the hypothesis stated objectively without value-laden words?
Yes No

f.   Is the direction of the relationship in the hypothesis clearly stated?
Yes No

g.   Is each of the hypotheses specific to one relationship so that each hypothesis can be either supported or not supported?
Yes No

2. *Hypothesis II:* There will be no difference in the time required by nursing assistants to complete dressing activities with cognitively impaired residents before and after implementing strategies to promote independence in dressing (SPID) (Beck et al, 1997).

a.   Is the hypothesis clearly stated in a declarative form?
Yes No

b.   Are the independent and dependent variables identified in the statement of the hypothesis?
Yes No

c.   Are the variables measurable or potentially measurable?
Yes No

d.   Is the hypothesis stated in such a way that it is testable?
Yes No

e.   Is the hypothesis stated objectively without value-laden words?
Yes No

f.   Is the direction of the relationship in the hypothesis clearly stated?
Yes No

g.   Is each of the hypotheses specific to one relationship so that each hypothesis can be either supported or not supported?
Yes No

Activity 7

You are designing a research study as part of the graduation requirements for your master's degree in nursing. In your personal time-line, you have committed 1 year (two 15-week semesters) to designing, obtaining human subjects approval, data collection, analysis, writing, and conducting the oral defense of this master's thesis. You would like to study the effect on patient outcomes on a cardiac unit based on the introduction of patient care technicians as team members to replace the primary care nursing model. The feasibility issues you will need to consider are time, availability of subjects, money, facilities and equipment, experience of the researcher, and ethical issues. For each of these issues described above, give your considered opinion as to why or why not this study would be feasible.

    a.   Time

    b.   Availability of subjects, money, facilities, and equipment

    c.   Experience of the researcher

    d.   Ethical issues

Another important element to consider when deciding to conduct research is to determine if this is a significant enough topic to study. Would the outcomes study proposed meet the criteria to be considered significant? Answer *yes* or *no* and then give the rationale underlying your choice.

Check your answers with those in Appendix A, Chapter 3.

Activity 8

How do you determine whether a sentence is a problem statement or a hypothesis?

Check your answers with those in Appendix A, Chapter 3.

Posttest

1. Choose the terms from the key provided that best describe items a through h. Write the appropriate abbreviation in the space provided. More than one abbreviation from the key may be used to describe each item.

   Key: RQ = Research question
   DH = Directional hypothesis
   NDH = Nondirectional hypothesis
   Hr = Research hypothesis
   Ho = Statistical hypothesis

   a. _____ There will be no change in self-rated body image among women in the three patient groups.

   b. _____ What is the relationship between organizational climate dimensions and job satisfaction of nurses in neonatal intensive care units?

   c. _____ The higher the perceived parental support, the lower the girls' general fearfulness.

   d. _____ There will be a significant difference in pre-post changes in cognitive development level between undergraduate nursing students who have completed a research course and those who have not.

   e. _____ The posttest mean of selected psychological variables for the experimental group will be lower than that of the control group.

   f. _____ There will be no association found between the level of social support and self-care health practices.

   g. _____ The educational preparation of a nurse (e.g., AA, diploma, BS) will affect his/her ability to conduct thorough patient interviews.

   h. _____ What is the level of postoperative infection following the use of clean tracheotomy care?

2. Fill in the blanks in the following sentences with the appropriate word or words from the list provided. Not all the words in the list will be used.

Research hypothesis   Null hypothesis
Predicts   Validity
Statistical hypothesis   Directional hypothesis
Testing   Declarative statement
Nondirectional hypothesis   Research question

a. The hypothesis is a vehicle for _____ the
    _____ of the assumptions of the theoretical framework of a
    research study.

b. A hypothesis transposes the question posed by the research problem into a
    _____ that _____ the relationship
    between two or more variables.

c. _____ hypotheses are more common than
    _____ hypotheses in studies that utilize deductive reasoning.

d. A _____ hypothesis is also known as the
    _____ hypothesis.

3. Review the Rudy et al (1995) article in Appendix C of the text.

a. Highlight the problem statement or hypothesis.

b. Is it a problem statement or hypothesis? Circle the correct answer.

c. List the variables being studied:

d. Critique the problem statement or hypothesis in the Rudy et al (1995) article focusing on the four criteria listed below. Circle your answer.

Criterion a: Clearly and unambiguously identifies the variables under consideration
Yes No

Criterion b: Clearly expresses the variables' relationship to each other
Yes No

Criteria c: Specifies the nature of the population being studied
Yes No

Criterion d: Implies the possibility of empirical testing
Yes No

e. Has the problem been placed within the context of an appropriate theoretical frame-work? If the answer is yes, list the framework described in the study.

4. Review the Draucker and Petrovic (1996) article in Appendix B of the text.

   a. Highlight the problem statement or hypothesis.

   b. Is it a problem statement or hypothesis? Circle the correct answer.

   c. List the variables being studied:

   d. Critique the problem statement or hypothesis in the Draucker and Petrovic (1996) article focusing on the four criteria listed below. Circle the correct answer.

   Criterion a: Clearly and unambiguously identifies the variables under consideration
   Yes   No

   Criterion b: Clearly expresses the variables' relationship to each other
   Yes   No

   Criterion c: Specifies the nature of the population being studied
   Yes   No

   Criterion d: Implies the possibility of empirical testing
   Yes   No

   e. Has the problem been placed within the context of an appropriate theoretical frame-work? If the answer is yes, list the framework described in the study.

The answers to the posttest are in the *Instructors' Resource Manual*.
Please check with your instructor for these answers.

References

Beck C et al: Improving dressing behavior in cognitively impaired nursing home residents, *Nurs Res* 46:126-131, 1997.

Bloom K, Trice L: The efficacy of individualized computerized testing in nursing education, *Computer Nurs* 15:82-88, 1997.

Brown J, Knapp T, Radke K: Sex, age, height, and weight as predictors of selected physiologic outcomes, *Nurs Res* 46:101-104, 1997.

Draucker B, Petrovic K: Healing of adult male survivors of childhood sexual abuse, *Image: J Nurs Schol* 28:325-330, 1996.

Goodwin S: The marital relationship and health in women with chronic fatigue and immune dysfunction syndrome: views of wives and husbands, *Nurs Res* 46:138-146, 1997.

Rudy EB et al: Patient outcomes for the chronically critically ill: special care unit versus intensive care unit, *Nurs Res* 44:324-331, 1995.

Ward SE, Berry PE, Misiewicz H: Concerns about analgesics among patients and family caregivers in a hospice setting, *Res Nurs Health* 19:205-211, 1996.

Wikblad K, Anderson B: A comparison of three wound dressings in patients undergoing heart surgery, *Nurs Res* 44:312-316, 1995.

Zerwic JJ, King KB, Wiasowicz GS: Perceptions of patients with cardiovascular disease about the causes of coronary artery disease, *Heart Lung* 26:92-98, 1997.

Literature Review

4

Mary Jo Gorney-Moreno

Introduction

The most common usage of the term review of the literature is to refer to that section of a research study in which the researcher describes the linkage between previously existing knowledge and the current study. Other research-related uses of a review of the literature are as follows:

1. Developing an overall impression of what research and clinical work has been done in a given area
2. Assisting in the clarification of the research problem
3. Polishing research design ideas
4. Finding possible data collection and data analysis strategies

This chapter will help you learn more about each of these uses of the literature to provide you with the basic information needed to decide whether a researcher has thoroughly reviewed the relevant literature, and used this review to its fullest potential.

Learning Outcomes

On completion of this chapter, the student should be able to do the following:

- Identify purposes of the literature review for research and nonresearch activities.
- Identify those paragraphs in any research study that constitute the literature review.
- Distinguish between primary and secondary sources.
- Differentiate between conceptual and data-based literature.
- Evaluate the degree to which relevant concepts and variables are discussed in the literature review.
- Compare the advantages and disadvantages of CD-ROM and Internet data bases with print data bases.
- Critically analyze the types of information available on the World Wide Web (WWW).

Activity 1

In the sentences listed below, fill in the blanks with the appropriate word or words from the italicized terms found in the following sentence:

The review of the literature is essential to the growth of nursing *theory*, *research*, *education*, and *practice*. In relation to these four concepts, a critical review of the literature does the following:

1. Reveals appropriate _____ questions for the discipline.

2. Provides the latest knowledge for _____.

3. Uncovers _____ findings that can lead to changes in clinical _____.

4. Uncovers new knowledge that can lead to the refinement of _____.

Check your answers with those in Appendix A, Chapter 4.

Activity 2

Listed below are examples of uses of the literature for research consumer purposes in educational and practice settings. Match the title of the research consumer in Column B with the description of activities in Column A. The titles will be used more than one time.

 You may want to review the AHCPR home page in Appendix B before answering this question.

Column A—Activities	Column B—Titles
1. _____ Develop ANA's social policy statement	a. Undergraduate student
2. _____ Implement research-based nursing interventions	b. Faculty
3. _____ Develop scholarly academic papers	c. Nurses in clinical setting
4. _____ Develop AHCPR's practice guidelines	d. Graduate students
5. _____ Develop research proposals for master's thesis	e. Governmental agencies
6. _____ Evaluate hospital CQI programs	f. Professional nursing organizations
7. _____ Revise curricula	

Check your answers with those in Appendix A, Chapter 4.

Activity 3

What follows is a list of terms and examples describing either conceptual or data-based literature. Put a *C* if the example describes conceptual literature, or a *D* if the example describes data-based literature. Refer to Tables 4-5 and 4-7 of the text for help.

1. _____ Published quantitative and qualitative studies

2. _____ Published articles or books discussing theories or concepts

3. _____ Unpublished abstracts of research studies from research conference

4. _____ Published studies in journal describing relationships between variables

5. _____ Teel C et al: Perspectives unifying symptom interpretation, *Image: J Nurs Schol* 29:175-181, 1997. The purpose was to introduce the symptom interpretation model (SIM) and facilitate understanding symptoms from an intrapersonal perspective. Theory derivation was used to develop SIM for understanding comparisons of known and new symptoms in a behavioral outcomes context.

6. _____ Oldham J, Howe T: The effectiveness of placebo muscle stimulation in quadriceps muscle rehabilitation: a preliminary evaluation, *Clin Effectiv Nurs* 1:25-30, 1997. The objective of this study was to evaluate the effect of placebo and "active" muscle stimulation in the rehabilitation of quadriceps muscle function in patients with osteoarthritis of the knee. All subjects were recruited from a waiting list for knee joint replacement.

Check your answers with those in Appendix A, Chapter 4.

Activity 4

Researchers who are also clinicians are interested in solving clinical problems—whether the solution is for immediate or future use. When faced with a problem in clinical practice, a clinician's common first thought is: What have others learned about this problem? The clinician usually goes first to the nursing literature to seek an answer to that question. List *five* nursing journals that publish reports or research studies that you as a clinician might study to find out more about a problem.

1.

2.

3.

4.

5.

Check your answers with those in Appendix A, Chapter 4.

Activity 5

The review of the literature is *usually* easy to find. In the abridged version of a research report, it is clearly labeled. Most frequently, one of the early sections of the report is labeled *Review of Literature* or *Relevant Literature* or some other comparable term. It may also be separated into a literature review section, and another section entitled *Conceptual Framework* that presents material on the theoretical or conceptual framework, which serves as the foundation for the study.

1. Examine the first two articles that are in the appendices of the text. What title is given to the literature review section?

   a. In Wikblad and Anderson?

   b. In Draucker and Petrovic?

   (*Note:* The length of the literature review section in a journal varies. A range from two paragraphs to several paragraphs is the most common.)

2. Does the literature review uncover gaps or inconsistencies in knowledge? If yes, state in your own words what gap or inconsistency is identified. If no, simply write "No."

   a. In Wikblad and Anderson?

   b. In Draucker and Petrovic?

3. Return to the Wikblad and Anderson article. Determine how recent the articles listed in the reference section are. There should be some from within 3 to 5 years and they should portray the development of the research over time. It should read like a good detective story, where at first there may be qualitative studies that attempt to identify which variables are important to this problem or paradigm. At some point you should also see researchers progressively analyze each of the variables, gradually narrowing and defining the scope of the problem, while others continue to look at the problem qualitatively. Do you see this in the literature and reference section of the Wikblad and Anderson article?

Circle either: Yes or No

Critique the currency of the references. Write the story you see in the reference section and as described in the review of the literature.

Check your answers with those in Appendix A, Chapter 4.

Activity 6

Sometimes it is difficult to understand the distinction between primary and secondary sources of information. There is a comparison that I have always found helpful. If you are considering giving a client an injection for pain, whose report would you feel most comfortable evaluating—the report of a family member or nurse's aide (i.e., secondary source) or the actual report by the client (i.e., primary source)? As a consumer of nursing research, you will also need to evaluate the credibility of research designs and reports based in part on whether they are generated from primary or secondary sources so that you know whether the information you are reading is a first-hand report or someone else's interpretation of the material.

1. The following words or phrases describe either primary or secondary sources. Put a *P* next to those describing primary and an *S* next to those describing secondary sources.

   a. _____ Summaries of research studies

   b. _____ First-hand accounts

   c. _____ Biographies

   d. _____ Textbooks

   e. _____ Patient records

   f. _____ Reports written by the researcher

   g. _____ Dissertations or master's theses

2. The best source for primary research studies is the WWW.
   True   False

3. You have a computer, fast modem, Web access provider, and WEB browser service at your home. You can now do your literature search in CINAHL OnLine without any additional cost.
   True   False

4. Information about CINAHL products and links to other nursing sources can be accessed at: http://www.cinahl.com/
   True   False

5. To use Internet Grateful Med, the user with Internet access and a MEDLARS account need only point a compatible WWW browser, such as Netscape Navigator, at the Internet Grateful Med URL: http://igm.nlm.nih.gov
   True   False

6. Which is the best data-base for a search of nursing literature? (See NLM home page in Appendix B.)
   A. MEDLINE
   B. CINAHL
   Why is one better than the other for nursing literature?

7. Print data-bases, such as CINAHL Print Index, must be used for literature searches of material before 1982.
   True   False

8. There is usually an extra charge for full text access to an article by fax or modem over the Internet from CINAHL (http://cinahl.com/) or another provider, such as Medical Matrix (http://www.medmatrix.org/info/medlinetable.html).
   True   False

9. The Sigma Theta Tau Law Registry of Nursing Research (see home page in Appendix B) and the Online Journal of Knowledge Synthesis for Nursing are available on the WEB for free.
   True   False

Check your answers with those in Appendix A, Chapter 4.

Activity 7

Below is a selected list of references from the Wikblad and Anderson article (see Appendix A in the textbook). Next to each, indicate whether the reference is conceptual (*C*) or data-based (*D*), and whether it is primary (*P*) or secondary (*S*).

Sometimes it is helpful to return to the text of the article and read the discussion of the reference; this may quickly inform you of the type of article that is referenced.

1. _____ _____   Bolton L, van Rijswijk L: Wound dressings: meeting clinical and biological needs, *Dermatology Nursing* 3:146-161, 1991.

2. _____ _____   Brennan PF, Hays BJ: The kappa statistic for establishing interrater reliability in the secondary analysis of qualitative clinical data, *Research in Nursing and Health* 15:153-158, 1992.

3. _____ _____   Cuzzell JZ: Choosing a wound dressing: a systematic approach, *AACN Clinical Issues in Critical Care Nursing* 1:566-577, 1990.

4. _____ _____   Feldman DL, Rogers A, Karpinski RH: A prospective trial comparing Biobrane, Duoderm and Xeroform for skin graft donor sites, *Surgery, Gynecology & Obstetrics* 173:1-5, 1991.

5. _____ _____ Hermans MH, Skillman NJ: Clinical benefit of a hydroactive dressing in closed surgical wounds, *Journal of ET Nursing* 20(2):68-72, 1993.

Check your answers with those in Appendix A, Chapter 4.

Activity 8

Many health care professionals and consumers now use the WWW to search for health care information. Before going on the WEB, develop a set of questions that you would like to use to critique the scientific merit of health care information obtained from the WWW. List at least *five* questions.

It may be helpful to recall what you have learned about the peer-review process before journal articles are accepted for publication, and to review the critiquing criteria in the textbook.

You may also want to review the home pages in Appendix B for an idea about what information is available on the World Wide Web.

1.

2.

3.

4.

5.

Check your answers with those in Appendix A, Chapter 4.

Posttest

1. Indicate whether the following are examples of primary (*P*) or secondary (*S*) sources.

a. _____ Pell J: Cardiac rehabilitation: a review of its effectiveness, *Cor Health Care* 1:8-17, 1997. This article reviews the published literature on the effectiveness of cardiac rehabilitation in terms of improving mortality, quality of life, and employment in those with myocardial infarction and stable angina pectoris.

b. _____ Zalon M: Pain in frail, elderly women after surgery, *Image: J Nurs Schol* 29:21-26, 1997. The purpose was to describe the lived experience of postoperative pain in frail, elderly women using Colaizzi's (1978) phenomenological approach.

2. Turn to the reference section in the Ward, Berry, and Misiewicz article (see Appendix D in the textbook), which is partially reproduced below. Next to each reference indicate whether it is conceptual (*C*), or data-based (*D*), and whether it is primary (*P*), or secondary (*S*).

   a. _____ _____ Ajzen I: The theory of planned behavior, *Organ Behav Hum Dec Process* 50:179-211, 1991.

   b. _____ _____ Ajzen I, Fishbein M: *Understanding attitudes and predicting social behavior*, Englewood Cliffs, NJ, 1980, Prentice-Hall.

   c. _____ _____ Berry P, Ward D: Barriers to pain management in hospice: a study of family caregivers, *Hospice J* 10(4):19-33, 1995.

   d. _____ _____ Breitbart W et al: *Patient-related barriers to pain management in AIDS*: Poster presented at the 13th Annual Meeting of the American Pain Society, Miami, FL, 1994.

3. Fill in the correct term.

   a. There are many (advantages; disadvantages) _____ for using computer data bases rather than just print data bases when doing a literature search.

   b. (Primary; Secondary) _____ sources are essential for literature reviews when designing a research proposal.

   c. The consumer of research should acquire the ability to (critically evaluate a review of the literature using critiquing criteria; use primary and secondary sources to write a literature review for a research study). _____

   d. To efficiently retrieve scholarly literature the nurse must both consult the reference librarian and (independently use e-mail; use computer CINAHL CD-ROM data bases).

_____

The answers to the posttest are in the *Instructor's Resource Manual*.
Please check with your instructor for these answers.

References

Draucker B, Petrovic K: Healing of adult male survivors of childhood sexual abuse, *Image: J Nurs Schol* 28:325-330, 1996.

Levine JR, Young ML, Reinhold A: *The internet for dummies*, Foster City, 1995, IDG Books Worldwide, Inc.

Oldham J, Howe T: The effectiveness of placebo muscle stimulation in quadriceps muscle rehabilitation: a preliminary evaluation, *Clin Effectiv Nurs* 1:25-30, 1997.

Pell J: Cardiac rehabilitation: a review of its effectiveness, *Cor Health Care* 1:8-17, 1997.

Pridham K: Mother's help seeking as care initiated in a social context, *Image: J Nurs Schol* 29:65-70, 1997.

Teel C et al: Perspectives unifying symptom interpretation, *Image: J Nurs Schol* 29:175-181, 1997.

Ward SE, Berry PE, Misiewicz H: Concerns about analgesics among patients and family caregivers in a hospice setting, *Res Nurs Health* 19:205-211, 1996.

Wikblad K, Anderson B: A comparison of three wound dressings in patients undergoing heart surgery, *Nurs Res* 44:312-316, 1995.

Zalon M: Pain in frail, elderly women after surgery, *Image: J Nurs Schol* 29:21-26, 1997.

Theoretical Framework

5

Kathleen Rose-Grippa

Introduction

It is not uncommon for the beginning consumer of research to find the theoretical part of a study to be the least favorite component. It tends to be heavily documented and is slow reading. It will not be long before you find it to be a very valuable aspect of any study. The theoretical framework of a study provides you with the opportunity to see the research problem through the eyes of the researcher. As the researcher develops and writes this section of the study, a window to his/her mind is opened. You get a glimpse of the way this particular researcher thinks about this particular problem. A critiquer's task is to listen respectfully to that person's perspective and then ask the following questions:

- How clearly do I understand the researcher's argument?
- Does the theoretical framework connect all of the pieces of the study?
- Can I see the relationship between the theoretical discussion and my clinical practice?

Most of the exercises in this chapter address the first question. Your ability to answer the second and third questions will improve as you complete the research course and as you build your clinical experiences.

Learning Objectives

On completion of this chapter, the student should be able to do the following:

- Discuss the following terms in relation to their distinguishing characteristics and value to a research study:
    a. Concept and construct
    b. Theoretical framework or theoretical rationale
    c. Conceptual definition
    d. Operational definition
    e. Variable
- Practice inductive and deductive thinking.
- Identify the major concepts in a given study.
- Trace the path of a variable from the introduction to the study through the theoretical component of given studies.
- Evaluate the relationship of a given theoretical framework to the relevant study and to clinical practice.

Activity 1

1. Jot down in your own words the defining characteristics of:

   Inductive thinking:

   Deductive thinking:

2. Play with these two kinds of thinking (i.e., inductive and deductive thinking) a bit before moving to clinical examples.

   a.   Imagine you are hungry. You look around for something to eat. You find a decorative tin labeled "candy" and decide that sounds good. You open the tin and see what looks like multicolored oval beads. Sure does not look like any candy you have ever seen before, but you trust the person who would be putting things in this tin so you decide to try them. Before long you notice yourself looking for the mottled pink, orange, yellow, and black ones because these taste good. You leave the mottled yellow, white, and reddish-brown ones alone because you do not like them.
   (Inductive; Deductive) _____ thinking would best describe your activity.

   b.   Sometime later you feel those old hunger pangs returning. This time that candy tin is empty. You want some more of those sweet multicolored oval beads. You start thinking, "Those beads were in the candy tin. They were sweet. There is a candy store around the corner. I bet the candy store will have these sweet beads. You walk to the candy store and discover that your thinking was correct. The candy store does have those sweet beads, and they call them jelly beans.
   (Inductive; Deductive) _____ describes your thinking style in this situation.

3. Now think about the concept of "pain." Think even more specifically about "headache pain." Picture several individuals, including yourself, when they are experiencing a headache. List your observations.

   Person #1   **Person#2**   **Person #3**   **Person #4**

Look across those observations. See any similarities? Maybe a creased forehead? Rubbing temples with fingertips? Rubbing forehead? Rubbing back of neck? Grumpy? Prefer less light? Reach for the over-the-counter pain medication? Grimaces?

Could you write a general statement about "signs of headache pain?" If "yes," please do so; if "no," jot down your thinking about why you are unable to write such a general statement.

Check your answers with those in Appendix A, Chapter 5.

Activity 2

As explained in the text, concepts are the building blocks of a study. The greater the ease with which you can identify concepts the easier it will become to analyze the theoretical framework of a given study. Once you can perform this analysis, you will be able to follow the line of logic from problem to conclusions.

1. Identify the concepts in each of the following excerpts from research:

    a. "A theoretical model was developed and tested to explain the effects of learned helplessness, self-esteem, and depression on the health practices of homeless women" (Flynn, 1997).

    b. ". . . was to examine the relationships among illness, uncertainty, stress, coping, and emotional well-being at the time of entry into a clinical drug trial" (Wineman et al, 1996).

    c. "As part of a larger study of the impact of a social support intervention on pregnancy outcome for lower-income African-American women. . ." (Bolla et al, 1996).

    d. ". . . to identify determinants of violent and nonviolent behavior among a group of vulnerable inner-city youths" (Powell, 1997).

e. ". . . prevalence and consequences of verbal abuse of staff nurses by physicians were examined in the context of Lazarus' stress-coping model" (Manderino and Berkey, 1997).

2. Now let's make things a bit more complex. Remember the definition of a "concept?" Sure you do! It is an abstraction. It is a term that creates an image of an idea or some notion that we humans want to share. Some concepts are more abstract than others. For example, "love" is more abstract than "table." Frequently, the terms concept and construct are used interchangeably. There is a subtle difference.

   a. Which term (beauty or nursing diagnosis) is a concept? Which is a construct?

   b. Think about the concept and construct in the previous question. How are they alike?

   c. How are they different?

3. Now it is your turn. Choose one concept from each of the five research examples in Item#1 of this activity. Write a definition of the chosen concept. Use your own words.

   a.

   b.

   c.

   d.

   e.

4. Compare your definition of the chosen concept with the definition of the same concept written by one of your peers. How close were you? Think about those similarities and differences. Assume the two of you were going to work as co-investigators on a study that addressed the chosen concept.

   a. What would you need to resolve?

b. Look one more time at those concepts. Do any of them more closely resemble a construct?

Check your answers with those in Appendix A, Chapter 5.

Activity 3

You have identified concepts, and you have written a definition of a concept. It is highly probable that the definition you wrote had more in common with a conceptual definition than with an operational definition. Operational definitions are a bit trickier. They need to be so clear that you, the reader, have no questions about what the researcher meant by each concept.

Think about the concept of "verbal abuse." What comes to mind when you hear that term (e.g., specific words such as swearing, put-downs, sarcasm; tone of voice, loudness of voice, frequency of abuse)? Verbal abuse was defined by Manderino and Berkey (1997) as the score on "the Verbal Abuse Scale (VAS)." They go on to explain that the Verbal Abuse Scale is "a recently developed 65-item self-report questionnaire (Manderino and Berkey, 1994), clearly defining 11 different forms of verbal abuse, thus permitting a focused exploration of the frequency and perceived stressfulness of the various manifestations of abuse." The 11 categories of verbal abuse are: ignoring, abusive anger, condescending, blocking/diverting, trivializing, abuse disguised as a joke, accusing/blaming, judging/criticizing, sexual harassment, discounting, and threatening.

Turn to the studies included in the four appendices of the textbook. Identify the conceptual and operational definitions in each of these studies. Do not expect every study to include both and do not be surprised if some definitions are implicit rather than explicit.

1. Wikblad and Anderson:

2. Draucker and Petrovic:

3. Rudy et al:

4. Ward, Berry, and Misiewicz:

Activity 4

Let's take a quick look at how theory, concepts, definitions, variables, and hypotheses fit together. There will be more detail about variables and hypotheses in a later chapter, so the focus here is more on an understanding of how they are based in theory.

1. Match the terms in Column B with the appropriate definition or example in Column A. Words in bold print in Column A indicate the element to be matched to a term. Items in Column B may be used more than once.

Column A   **Column B**

a. _____ **"Fatigue symptoms were measured using the**   1. Variable
          Modified Fatigue Symptoms Checklist (MFSC),
          a list of 30 symptoms of fatigue. Scores range   2. Hypothesis
          from zero (no fatigue symptoms) to 30 symptoms
          (maximum fatigue)." (Milligan, Flenniken, and   3. Construct
          Pugh, 1996)
                                                                 4. Operational definition
b. _____ ". . . **stress** and **empowerment** were used to guide
          this study." (Kendra, 1996)   5. Concept

c. _____ "Serenity is viewed as a **learned, positive emotion** 6. Conceptual definition
          of inner peace that can be sustained . . . that
          decreases perceived stress and improves physical
          and emotional health." (Roberts and Whall, 1996)

d. _____ Older (i.e., **more than 35 years old**) first-time mothers (Reese and Harkless, 1996)

e. _____ **Clinical decision-making**

f. _____ **Quality of life**

g. _____ "Acute confusion is a transient syndrome characterized primarily by **abnormali-
          ties in attention and cognition,** but **disordered psychomotor behavior, sleep-
          wake disturbance, and autonomic nervous system disturbances** are not
          uncommon." (Neelon et al, 1996)

h. _____ "Are there **breathing pattern changes** from test to test or from the beginning to
          the end of the test?" (Hopp et al, 1996)

i. _____ "The **combination of injury experience, knowledge, demographic, health
          beliefs, and social influence variables will predict home hazard
          accessibility."** (Russell and Champion, 1996)

2. This exercise allows you the opportunity to use all of the thinking you have done so far in tracing a variable from the introduction of a study through the theoretical rationale of that same study. Turn to Appendix A of the textbook and read the first part of the Wikblad and Anderson study. Read from the beginning of the study (including the title) to the section entitled "Method." Do not read the methods section.

    a.   Name the main variable in this study (read the title closely for this information):

    b.   Read the next six paragraphs and summarize in one sentence per paragraph what you learned about wound dressings.

        i.

        ii.

        iii.

        iv.

        v.

        vi.

    c.   What type of reasoning is operating in this study?

    d.   Were hypotheses developed for this study?

    e.   Would you describe the theoretical rationale for this study as:

        _____ A theoretical framework   _____ A theory

        _____ A conceptual model   _____ None of the above

    f.   What is the clinical concern that is the basis of this study?

Check your answers with those in Appendix A, Chapter 5.

Activity 5

Use the grid that follows and critique the theoretical component of the four studies found in the appendices of the text. In the grid, identify the study that satisfies that particular criterion, that is, use *W/A* for Widblad and Anderson, *D* for Drauker and Petrovic, *R* for Rudy et al, and *W/B* for Ward, Berry, and Misiewicz.

CRITIQUING GRID

	Well Done	OK	Needs Help	Not Applicable
1. Theoretical rationale was clearly identified (Could I find it?)				
2. The information in the theoretical component matches what the researchers are studying				
3. Concepts: a. Conceptual definition(s) found b. Conceptual definition(s) clear c. Operational definition(s) found d. Operational definition(s) clear				
4. Enough literature was reviewed: a. For an expert in the area b. For a nurse with some knowledge c. For a nurse reading outside of area of specialty or interest				
5. Thinking of researcher: a. Can be followed through theoretical material to hypotheses or questions b. Makes sense				
6. Relationships among propositions clearly stated				
7. Theory: a. Borrowed b. Concepts/data related to nursing				
8. Findings related back to theoretical base. I can find each concept from the theory section discussed in the "Results" section of the report				

Posttest

1. List three reasons supporting the importance of the theoretical rationale of a study.

   a.

   b.

   c.

2. Read each statement. Decide if the statement is true or false. Mark with a *T* if the statement is true and with an *F* if the statement is false. Rewrite the false statements to make them true statements.

   a. _____ "Caregiving" is an example of a concept that is so clearly understood there is no need for it to be operationally defined in a research study.

   b. _____ The following definition is an example of a conceptual definition: "The Beck Dressing Performance Scale (BDPS) (Beck, 1988) was used to measure the major dependent variable, the level of caregiver assistance provided during dressing. The dressing function is broken down into 42 discrete component steps for males and 45 for females. A trained rater assigns each step of the dressing activity a score of 0 (independent) to 7 (complete dependence) based on the amount of assistance required to complete each step. Higher scores indicate greater dependence." (Beck et al, 1997)

   c. _____ The words in bold in the following phrase are the name of a construct: ". . . define **a professional practice model (PPM)** as a system that supports registered nurse control over the delivery of nursing care and the environment in which care is delivered." (Hoffart and Woods, 1997)

   d. _____ The following is an example of a conceptual definition: "Although there is no standard definition of social support, there seems to be general acceptance of some basic typologies. House, Umberson, and Landis (1988) defined social support as positive dimensions of relationships that may promote health and buffer stress." (Bolla et al, 1996)

   e. _____ The following is a sketch of a concept: ". . . verbal abuse was defined as verbal behaviors that are perceived as humiliating, degrading, and/or disrespectful. "Because verbally abusive encounters potentially can be stressful, it seemed appropriate to address this issue within the framework of a model of stress . . . the major tenet of this model [sic: Lazarus' transactional model of stress coping] is that stress occurs in the face of perceived demands that tax or exceed the perceived coping resources of the person." (Manderino and Berkey, 1997)

   Answers to the posttest are in the *Instructor's Resource Manual*.
   Please check with your instructor for these answers.

References

Beck C et al: Improving dressing behavior in cognitively impaired nursing home residents, *Nurs Res* 46(3):126-132, 1997.

Bolla CD et al: Social support as a road map and vehicle: an analysis of data from focus group interviews with a group of African American women, *Public Health Nurs* 13(5):331-336, 1996.

Flynn L: The health practices of homeless women: a causal model, *Nurs Res* 46(2):72-77, 1997.

Hoffart N, Woods CQ: Elements of a nursing professional practice model, *J Prof Nurs* 12(6):354-364, 1997

Hopp LJ et al: Incremental threshold loading in patients with chronic obstructive pulmonary disease, *Nurs Res* 45(4):196-202, 1996.

Kendra MA: Perception of risk by home health care administrators and field workers, *Public Health Nurs* 13(6):386-393, 1996.

Manderino MA, Berkey N: Verbal abuse of staff nurses by physicians, *J Prof Nurs* 13(1):48-55, 1997.

Milligan RA, Flenniken PM, Pugh LC: Positioning intervention to minimize fatigue in breast-feeding women, *Appl Nurs Res* 9(2):67-70, 1996.

Neelon VJ et al: The Neecham confusion scale: construction, validation, and clinical testing, *Nurs Res* 45(6):324-330, 1996.

Powell KB: Correlates of violent and nonviolent behavior among vulnerable inner-city youths, *Family Comm Health* 20(2):38-47, 1997.

Reese SM, Harkless G: Clinical methods: divergent themes in maternal experience in women older than 35 years of age, *Appl Nurs Res* 9(3):148-153, 1996.

Roberts KT, Whall A: Serenity as a goal for nursing practice, *Image: J Nurs Schol* 28(4):359-364, 1996.

Russell KM, Champion VL: Health beliefs and social influence in home safety practice of mothers with preschool children, *Image: J Nurs Schol* 28(1):59-64, 1996.

Wineman NM et al: Relationships among illness uncertainty, stress, coping, and emotional well-being at entry into a clinical drug trial, *Appl Nurs Res* 9(2):53-60, 1996.

Introduction to Design

Ann Marttinen Doordan

Introduction

The term *research design* is used to describe the overall plan of a particular study. The design is the researcher's plan for answering specific research questions in the most accurate and efficient way possible. The design ties together the present research problem, the knowledge of the past, and the implications for the future. Thus the choice of a design reflects the researcher's experience, expertise, knowledge, and biases.

Learning Outcomes

On completion of this chapter, the student should be able to do the following:
- Identify the major components of a research design.
- Identify threats to internal validity.
- Identify threats to external validity.
- State the relationship between the research design and internal and external validity.
- Critically analyze the strengths and limitations of the chosen design for a specific study.

Activity 1

Match the definition of the terms in column A with the research design terms in column B. Each term is used no more than once and not all terms will be used. Check the glossary for help with terms.

Column A	Column B
1. _____ A blueprint for conducting a research study.	a. External validity
2. _____ All parts of a study follow logically from the problem statement.	b. Internal validity
	c. Accuracy
3. _____ Methods to keep the study conditions constant during the study.	d. Research design
4. _____ Consideration whether the study is possible and practical to conduct.	e. Control
	f. Random sampling
5. _____ A sample of subjects similar to one another.	g. Feasibility
6. _____ Process to ensure every subject has an equal chance of being selected.	h. Homogenous sampling
7. _____ Degree to which a research study is consistent within itself.	i. Objectivity
8. _____ Degree to which the study results can be applied to the larger population.	

Check your answers with those in Appendix A, Chapter 6.

Activity 2

For each of the following situations identify the type of threat to internal validity from the following list. Then explain the reason this is a problem, and suggest how this problem can be corrected.

> History
> Instrumentation
> Maturation
> Mortality
> Selection bias
> Testing

1. Nurses on a maternity unit want to study the effect of a new hospital-based teaching program on mothers' confidence in caring for their newborn infants. The researchers mail out a survey one month after discharge.

2. In a study of the results of a hypertension teaching program conducted at a senior center, the blood pressures taken by volunteers using their personal equipment were compared before and after the program.

3. A major increase in cigarette taxes occurs during a one-year follow-up study of the impact of a smoking cessation program.

4. The smoking cessation rates of an experimental group consisting of volunteers for a smoking cessation program were compared with the results of a control group of persons who wanted to quit on their own without a special program.

5. Thirty percent of the subjects dropped out of an experimental study of the effect of a job training program on employment for homeless women. Over 90% of the dropouts were single homeless women with at least two preschool children, while the majority of subjects successfully completing the program had no preschool children.

6. The researcher tested the effectiveness of a new method of teaching drug dosage and solution calculations to nursing students using a standardized calculation exam at the beginning, midpoint, and end of a 2-week course.

Check your answers with those in Appendix A, Chapter 6.

Activity 3

The term *research design* is an all-encompassing term for the overall plan to answer the research questions, including the method and specific plans to control other factors that could influence the results of the study.

1. To become acquainted with the major elements in the design of a study, read the study comparing wound dressings by Wikblad and Anderson in Appendix A in the textbook and answer the following questions:

    a. What was the setting for the study?

    b. Who were the subjects?

    c. How was the sample selected?

    d. What information was missing?

    e. Was this a homogenous sample?

    f. How were variables measured and constancy maintained?

    g. Which group served as the control group?

    Check your answers with those in Appendix A, Chapter 6.

Activity 4

Use the critiquing criteria in Chapter 6 to critique the research design of the Wikblad and Anderson study in Appendix A of the textbook. (Explain your answers.)

1. Is the design appropriate?

2. Is the control consistent with the research design?

3. Is the economy reflected?

4. Does the design logically flow from problem, framework, literature review, and hypothesis?

5. What are the threats to internal validity?

6. What are the controls for threats to internal validity?

7. What are the threats to external validity?

8. What are the controls for threats to external validity?

Check your answers with those in Appendix A, Chapter 6.

Posttest

1. Review the Rudy et al (1995) study, *Patient Outcomes for the Chronically Critically Ill: Special Care Unit Versus Intensive Care Unit*, in Appendix C of the textbook. Briefly assess the major components of the research design.

   a. What is the purpose of the study?

   b. What is the setting for the study?

   c. Who are the subjects?

   d. How is the sample selected?

   e. What is the research treatment?

   f. How do the researchers attempt to control elements affecting the results of the study?

2. Fill in the blanks by selecting from the following list of terms. Not all terms will be used.

Constancy   Mortality
Control   Internal validity
Feasibility   External validity
Selection bias   Accuracy
Reliability   History
Maturation

a. _____ is used to hold steady the conditions of the study.

b. _____ is used to describe that all aspects of a study logically follow from the problem statement.

c. The believability between this study and the world at large is known as _____.

d. The developmental, biological, or psychological processes known as _____ operate within a person over time and may influence the results of a study.

e. Time, subject availability, equipment, money, experience, and ethics are factors influencing the _____ of a study.

f. Selection bias, mortality, maturation, instrumentation, testing, and history influence the _____ of a study.

g. Voluntary, rather than random, assignment to an experimental or control condition creates a situation known as _____

The answers to the posttest are in the *Instructor's Resource Manual*.
Please check with your instructor for these answers.

References

Rudy EB et al: Patient outcomes for the chronically critically ill: special care unit versus intensive care unit, *Nurs Res* 44:324-331, 1995.

Wikblad K, Anderson B: A comparison of three wound dressings in patients undergoing heart surgery, *Nurs Res* 44:312-316, 1995.

Experimental and Quasiexperimental Designs 7

Ann Marttinen Doordan

Introduction

This chapter contains exercises for two categories of design: experimental and quasi-experimental. These types of designs allow researchers to test the effects of nursing actions and make statements about cause-effect relationships. Therefore, they can be very helpful in testing solutions to nursing practice problems. However, a researcher chooses the design that allows a given situation or problem to be studied in the most accurate and effective way possible. Thus, not all problems are amenable to immediate study by these two types of designs. Rather, the choice of design is dependent on the development of knowledge relevant to the problem, plus the researcher's knowledge, experience, expertise, preferences, and resources.

Learning Outcomes

On completion of this chapter, the student should be able to do the following:
- Identify the components of experimental and quasiexperimental research designs.
- Compare and contrast experimental and quasiexperimental research designs.
- Critique the type of design used in experimental, quasiexperimental, and program evaluation studies.
- Critique the application potential of the findings of specific experimental and quasiexperimental studies.

Activity 1

Fill in the blank for each of the following descriptions with a term selected from the list of types of experimental and quasiexperimental designs. Each term is used only once and not all terms may be used.
Consult the glossary for assistance with definition of terms.

> True experiment
> Solomon four-group
> After-only experiment
> Nonequivalent control group
> After-only nonequivalent control group
> Time series
> Evaluation research

1. The type of design that has two groups identical to the true experimental design plus an experimental after-group and a control after-group is known as a(n) _____ design.

2. A research approach used when only one group is available to study for trends over a longer period of time is called a(n) _____ design.

3. The _____ design is also known as the posttest only control group design in which neither the experimental group nor the control group is pretested.

4. If a researcher wants to compare results obtained from an experimental group with a control group, but was unable to conduct pretests or to randomly assign subjects to groups, the study would be known as a(n) _____ design.

5. The _____ design includes three properties: randomization, control, and manipulation.

6. When subjects are unable to be randomly assigned into experimental and control groups but are able to be pretested and posttested, the design is known as a(n) _____ design.

Check your answers with those in Appendix A, Chapter 7.

Activity 2

Review the study by Wikblad and Anderson (1995), *A Comparison of Three Wound Dressings in Patients Undergoing Heart Surgery*, found in Appendix A of the textbook, then answer the following questions.

1. The classic experiment has three properties: randomization, control, and manipulation of variables. How were each of these conditions applied in this study?

   a. Randomization

   b. Control

   c. Manipulation

2. How does this study handle potential threats to internal validity, such as maturation, history, or selection bias?

3. List the implications of this study for nursing practice.

4. What difference would there be in interpreting the results if the researcher had not used randomization?

5. What difference would there be in interpreting the results if the researcher had not used a control group?

Check your answers with those in Appendix A, Chapter 7.

Activity 3

The education department in a large hospital wants to test a program to educate and change nurses attitudes regarding pain management. They have a questionnaire that measures nurses' knowledge and attitudes about pain. Your responsibility is to design a study to examine the outcome of this intervention program.

1. You decide to use a Solomon four-group design. Complete the chart below with an X to indicate which of the four groups receive the pretest and posttest pain questionnaire and which receive the experimental teaching program.

	Pretest	Teaching	Posttest
Group A	_____	_____	_____
Group B	_____	_____	_____
Group C	_____	_____	_____
Group D	_____	_____	_____

2. How would you assign nurses to each of the four groups?

3. What would you use as a pretest for the groups receiving the pretest?

4. What is the experimental treatment?

5. What is the outcome measure for each group?

6. Based on your reading, for what types of issues is this design particularly effective?

7. What is the major advantage for this type of design?

8. What is a disadvantage for this type of design?

Check your answers with those in Appendix A, Chapter 7.

Activity 4

For each of the following descriptions of experimental or quasiexperimental studies, identify the type of design used in the study and the advantages and disadvantages of this design.

1. The purpose of this study was to evaluate the relationship of pulmonary rehabilitation to psychosocial adjustment to COPD and use of healthcare services. Adjustment scores and use of healthcare services were compared for 13 individuals who had not had formal pulmonary rehabilitation and 17 individuals who had completed a formal pulmonary rehabilitation program. (Lewis and Bell, 1995).

   a.   What type of design was used?

   b.   What are the advantages of this design?

   c.   What are the disadvantages of this design?

2. The effectiveness of a special intervention to help patients decrease dietary fat intake, reduce smoking, and increase exercise was conducted with 138 women who had coronary artery bypass surgery. Subjects were randomly assigned into special intervention or usual care groups. Risk factors and lifestyle behaviors were measured at baseline and 1 year after surgery (Allen, 1996).

   a.   What type of design was used?

   b.   What are the advantages of this design?

   c.   What are the disadvantages of this design?

3. The performance of 56 students in an accelerated baccalaureate nursing program for college graduates and a traditional baccalaureate nursing program were compared. Students in each group completed the pretest and the posttest on nursing performance (McDonald, 1995).

   a.   What type of design was used?

   b.   What are the advantages of this design?

   c.   What are the disadvantages of this design?

4. The purpose of the study was to compare behavioral and interactional differences in irritable and nonirritable infants. Forty infants and their mothers were assessed every 3 weeks from 4 weeks to 16 weeks of age (Keefe et al, 1996).

   a.   What type of design was used?

   b.   What are the advantages of this design?

   c.   What are the disadvantages of this design?

   Check your answers with those in Appendix A, Chapter 7.

Activity 5

1. You may be questioning why anyone would use a quasiexperimental design if an experimental design has the advantage of being so much stronger in detecting cause and effect relationships and enables the researcher to generalize the results to a wider population. In what instances might it be advantageous to use a quasiexperimental design?

2. What must the researcher do in order to generalize the findings from a quasiexperimental research study?

3. What must a clinician do before application of research findings into practice?

Posttest

1. Identify whether the following studies are experimental or quasiexperimental. Use the abbreviations from the key provided.

Key: E = Experimental
       Q = Quasiexperimental

a. _____ Fifty teen mothers are randomly assigned into an experimental parenting support group and a regular support group. Before the program and at the end of the 3-month program, mother-child interaction patterns are compared between the two groups.

b. _____ Patients on two separate units are given a patient satisfaction with care questionnaire to complete at the end of their first hospital day and on the day of discharge. The patients on one unit receive care directed by a nurse case manager, and the patients on the other unit receive care from the usual rotation of nurses. Patient satisfaction scores are compared.

c. _____ Students are randomly assigned to two groups. One group receives an experimental independent study program and the other receives the usual classroom instruction. Both groups receive the same posttest to evaluate learning.

d. _____ A study was conducted to compare the effectiveness of a music relaxation program with silent relaxation on lowering blood pressure ratings. Subjects were randomly assigned into groups and blood pressures were measured before, during, and immediately after the relaxation exercises.

e. _____ Reading and language development skills were compared between a group of children with chronic otitis media and a group of children without a history of ear problems.

2. Identify the type of experimental or quasiexperimental design for each of the following examples. Use the numbers from the key provided.

Key: 1 = After-only
       2 = After-only nonequivalent control group
       3 = True experiment
       4 = Nonequivalent control group
       5 = Time series
       6 = Solomon four-group

a. _____ Nurses are randomly assigned to a new self-study program or the usual ECG teaching program. Knowledge of ECGs is tested before and after the program for both groups.

b. _____ Babies who tested positive on toxicology screening at birth are randomly assigned into groups to either receive routine care or to receive a special public health nurse intervention program. Health outcomes are tested and compared at 6 months.

c. _____ A school nurse clinic is set up at one school. Health care outcomes are measured at the end of a year from that school and compared with health outcomes at a comparable school that does not have a clinic.

d. _____ Diabetic patients were randomly assigned to either one of two control groups receiving routine home health care or to one of two groups with a new diabetic teaching program. Patients in one of the control groups and in one of the teaching groups took a test of diabetic knowledge as soon as they were assigned to a group. Patients in the other two groups were not pretested. All patients completed a posttest at the conclusion of the 3-week program.

e. _____ A new peer AIDS prevention program was implemented in one high school. A second high school without the program served as a control group. An AIDS knowledge test was administered at both schools before and after the program was completed.

f. _____ Trends in patient falls were summarized each week one year before and for the first year after implementation of a new hospital-based quality assurance program.

The answers to the posttest are in the *Instructor's Resource Manual*.
Please check with your instructor for these answers.

References

Allen JK: Coronary risk factor modification in women after coronary artery bypass surgery, *Nurs Res* 45:260-265, 1996.

Keefe MR et al: A longitudinal comparison of irritable and nonirritable infants, *Nurs Res* 45:4-9, 1996.

Lewis D, Bell SK: Pulmonary rehabilitation, psychosocial adjustment, and use of healthcare services, *Rehab Nurs* 20:102-107, 1995.

McDonald WK: Comparison of performance of students in an accelerated baccalaureate nursing program for college graduates and a traditional nursing program, *J Nurs Educ* 34:123-127, 1995.

Wikblad K, Anderson B: A comparison of three wound dressings in patients undergoing heart surgery, *Nurs Res* 44:312-316, 1995.

Nonexperimental Designs

Mary Jo Gorney-Moreno

Introduction

Nonexperimental designs can provide extensive amounts of data that can help fill in the gaps found in nursing research. These designs help us clarify, see the real world, and assess relationships between variables, and they can provide clues to direct future, more controlled research. In this way experimental and nonexperimental designs complement each other. Each provides necessary components of our lives. Nonexperimental designs allow us to discover some of the territory of nursing knowledge before trying to rearrange parts of it. It can be the basis on which knowledge is built and further refined with experimental research.

Learning Outcomes

On completion of this chapter, the student should be able to do the following:
- Identify the type of nonexperimental design used in a given study when provided the relevant sentences from the abstract or report of the research.
- Identify advantages and disadvantages of using nonexperimental designs for given problems.
- List the most appropriate type of nonexperimental design given specific research situations.
- Critique the use of nonexperimental designs for specific studies.

Activity 1

Determine an answer for each of the following items. Once you have an answer, study the diagram to find each answer. The words will always be in a straight-line. They may be read up or down, left to right, right to left, or diagonally. When you find one of the words, draw a circle around it. Any single letter may be used in more than one word; however, all of the letters will not be used. There are no spaces or hyphens between the words in the puzzle; therefore, if it is a multiword answer, link the letters together as if it is all one word. Some terms will be used more than once to fill in the blanks in the statements.

```
L O N G I T U D I N A L D M E
C I S P U E Q W H X O I Y H X
C R F L G Y Q E R C X E C G P
U W O L Z S B Q F H V O H H O
N T L S C I S Z A R R O I U S
L G T R S D L D U R Z L D O T
U E I O I S Q S E D L Y W O F
I U W S J J E L O S Y U H I A
G T D K X O A C I E M D I I C
Q W R E E T O K T T E S T A T
A S A M I K E N B I B H U L O
D U O O K L H N P H O B Z V F
M C N G U L U E O L Y N R K C
K A M F G U P Q S B Z L A H T
L W J F V N E W J S W L E L Y
```

1. This type is better known for breadth of data collected than depth.

2. A major disadvantage is the length of time needed for data collection.

3. The main question is whether or not variables covary.

4. This words means *after the fact*.

5. This eliminates the confounding variable of maturation.

6. This quantifies the magnitude and direction of a relationship.

7. Collects data from the same group at several points in time.

8. Can be surprisingly accurate if the sample is representative.

9. Uses data from one point in time.

10. This is based on two or more naturally occuring groups with different conditions of the presumed independent variable.

Check your answers with those in Appendix A, Chapter 8.

Activity 2

Listed below are a series of advantages and disadvantages for various types of nonexperimental designs. For each type of design pick at least one advantage (A) and one disadvantage (D) from the list that accurately describes a quality of the design. Then insert the A or D and the appropriate number in the list below.

	Advantages	Disadvantages
Correlation studies	_____	_____
Cross-sectional	_____	_____
Descriptive/exploratory	_____	_____
Ex post facto	_____	_____
Longitudinal	_____	_____
Prediction studies	_____	_____
Prospective	_____	_____
Retrospective	_____	_____
Survey	_____	_____

Advantages

A1 A great deal of information can be economically obtained from a large population.
A2 Ability to assess changes in the variables of interest over time.
A3 Explores relationship between variables that are inherently not manipulable.
A4 Offers a higher level of control than a correlational study.
A5 They facilitate intelligent decision making by using objective criteria to guide process.
A6 Each subject is followed separately and serves as his/her own control.
A7 Stronger than retrospective studies because of the degree of control on extraneous variables.

Disadvantages

D1 The inability to draw a causal linkage between two variables.
D2 An alternative hypothesis could be the reason for the relationships.
D3 The researcher is unable to manipulate the variables of interest.
D4 The researcher is unable to determine a causal relationship between variables because of lack of manipulation, control, and randomization.
D5 The information obtained tends to be superficial.
D6 The researcher must know sampling techniques, questionnaire construction, interviewing, and data analysis.
D7 No randomization in sampling because studying preexisting groups.
D8 Internal validity threats, such as testing and mortality, are present.

Check your answers with those in Appendix A, Chapter 8.

Activity 3

Each of the following are excerpts from nonexperimental studies. For each example, determine the type of design used from the list provided. Not all designs are used as examples, and designs will be used more than one time.

C   Correlation studies
CS   Cross-sectional
D/E/S   Descriptive/exploratory/survey studies
E   Ex post facto
L   Longitudinal
M   Methodological
MA   Metaanalysis
PS   Prediction studies
P   Prospective
R   Retrospective

Remember, some studies use more than one type of nonexperimental design.

1. "Historical evidence shows women's attempts to achieve the current societally mandated esthetic ideals. Although a sociocultural impact is generally acknowledged, no measurement instrument has been developed to empirically confirm it. A questionnaire measuring the respondent's recognition and acceptance of the prevailing societal message was developed and validated in a series of 3 studies." (Heinberg L, Thompson JK, and Stormer S, 1995)
Type of design:

2. The objective of Sherman's 1996 study was to: "Use Rogers' (1992) framework of the science of unitary human beings to examine relationships among spirituality, perceived social support, death anxiety, and nurses' willingness to care for AIDS patients." The data collection instruments used were: Spiritual Orientation Inventory, the Personal Resource Questionnaire-85, the Templer Death Anxiety Scale, and the Willingness to Care for AIDS Patients Instrument. The findings: "Willingness to care for AIDS patients was positively correlated with spirituality and perceived social support, and negatively correlated with death anxiety." (Sherman, 1996)
Type of design:

3. "The growth of information technology systems associated with the organizational reforms of the British Health Service has given rise to a need to understand nurses' attitudes toward computerization. Several studies in the United States have identified various factors that influence nurses' computer-related attitudes but such studies in the United Kingdom are rare. This study sampled 208 nurses in a general hospital of approximately 500 beds, and measured their computer-related attitudes using Stronge and Brodth's questionnaire . . . A total of 430 questionnaires were distributed to all nursing staff in the study hospital of which 208 were returned, representing a response rate of 48.4%." (Simpson and Kenrick, 1997)
Type of design:

4. "This article assessed the effectiveness of different treatments for bulimia nervosa by screening 400 studies published from 1987 through July 1993. Nineteen independent studies with a total of 1,015 subjects with 11 treatment types, and 316 subject in 11 control groups fulfilled these criteria." (McGown A and Whitbread J, 1996)
Type of design:

5. "The purpose of this study was to examine the health behaviors of nursing students as they entered and again as they completed their baccalaureate nursing education to see what lifestyle changes occurred as students were exposed to a healthcare curriculum." The procedure followed was that of the Health Promoting Lifestyle Profile, a 48-item instrument administered to students during the first and again during the last semester of their nursing program. (Riordan and Washburn, 1997)
Type of design:

6. The purpose was: ". . . to survey paternal worries, concerns, stresses, or problems and the type of support received by men whose partners were prescribed bed rest at home, or in the hospital or both . . . A national subsample of 59 men whose mates had been on pregnancy bed rest were randomly selected in 1995 from a nonrandom select sample of individuals who had contacted a bed-rest support group (Sidelines) for information. The mean total length of bedrest was 92.1 days . . . The majority of the women were on both home and hospital bed rest (n = 36, 61%), while 21 were solely on home bed rest, and two were only on hospital bed rest; 53% had been on bed rest within the last year and all but 17% had been on bed rest within the last 2 years . . ." (Maloni and Ponder, 1997)
Type of design:

Check your answer with those in Appendix A, Chapter 8

Activity 4

Use the critiquing criteria from the chapter to analyze the following excerpt from a study.
In a 1997 article by Mohr, her objective was: "This study is the context portion of a larger study that described the experience of 30 nurses in Texas, USA, who worked in for-profit psychiatric hospitals during a documented period of corporate deviance. The objective of the contextual portion was to describe the major findings in 1991-1992 of investigating agencies that probed the scandal." The sample consisted of more than 1,240 pages and 40 hours of corporate records obtained under subpoena, in addition to written and oral testimony before the USA House Select Committee on Children, Youth, and Families.

1. Type of design:

The findings were four themes: insurance games, dumping patients, patient abuse, and playing with the language.
The conclusions "Organizational deviance may become more widespread in profit-driven sys-

tems of care. Lobbying for whistleblower protection, collective advocacy, and creative educational reforms are used" are presented in the frontpiece of the article. However, under the *Discussion and Recommendations* section, the author states: "As suggested by social scientists, research can serve as the basis for reflection, critique and action . . . For example, because nurses are professionals who have a special contract with the public and are concerned with health teaching and promotion, they might implement counter-hegemonic activity by collective advocacy and criticizing information disortion."

2. Does the research go beyond the relational parameters of the findings and erroneously infer cause-and-effect relationships between the variables?

   Circle: Yes   No   (If yes, explain below.)

   Check your answers with those in Appendix A, Chapter 8

 # Activity 5

Review the Critical Thinking Decision Path: Design Choice found in the textbook. If you wanted to test a relationship between two variables in the past such as the incidence of reported back injuries of nurses working in a newborn nursery compared to that of nurses working in long-term care:

Which design would you use?

Check your answers with those in Appendix A, Chapter 8

Posttest

Choose from among the following words to complete the posttest. Each word may only be used one time; however, this list duplicates some words because they appear in more than one answer.

Retrospective	Longitudinal	Survey	Descriptive
Exploratory	Interrelational	Correlational	Ex post facto
Retrospective	Cross sectional	Retrospective	Prospective
Cross sectional	Longitudinal	Prospective	

1. _____ is the broadest category of nonexperimental design.

2. It can be further classified as _____ and _____.

3. The second major category of nonexperimental design according to LoBiondo-Wood and Haber is _____

4. The researcher is using _____ design when examining the relationship between two or more variables.

5. _____ designs have many similarities to quasiexperimental designs.

6. _____ design used in epidemiological work is similar to ex post facto.

7. LoBiondo-Woods and Haber discuss the following *four* types of developmental studies:

   a.

   b.

   c.

   d.

8. _____ studies data at one point in time while _____ collects data from the same group at different points in time.

9. A(n) _____ study looks at presumed causes and moves forward in time to presumed effects.

10. The researcher is using a(n) _____ design if he/she is trying to link present events to events that have occurred in the past.

11. The following is an excerpt from a nonexperimental study. Determine the type of design used and insert its name in the space provided.

    Remember, some studies use more than one type of nonexperimental design.

    "This empirical study explored the attitudes and participation of registered nurses (RNs) in New South Wales (NSW), Australia in continuing professional education . . . A 25-item questionnaire was developed and mailed to a random sample of 500 RNs currently licensed to practice within NSW. Respondent anonymity was assured by having the Nurses Registration Board generate the random sample and undertake the mailing." (Kersaitis, 1997).

    Type of design:

12. Review the Ward, Berry, and Misiewicz (1996) *Concerns about Analgesics Among Patients and Family Caregivers in a Hospice Setting* (see Appendix D in the textbook).

Answer the following questions based on this article.

a. Type of design

Variables being studied

Name one advantage and one disadvantage of this design in relation to this specific study.

b. Advantage

c. Disadvantage

 d. Does the researcher present the findings in a manner that is incongruent with the utilized design?

e. Does the research go beyond the relational parameters of the findings and erroneously infer cause-and-effect relationships between the variables?

f. How does the author deal with the limitations of the study?

The answers to the posttest are in the *Instructor's Resource Manual*.
Please check with your instructor for these answers.

References

Heinberg LJ, Thompson JK, Storner S: Development and validation of the sociocultural attitudes towards appearance questionnaire, *Inter J Eat Dis* 17:81-89, 1995.

Kersaitis C: Attitudes and participation of registered nurses in continuing professional education in New South Wales, Australia, *J Contin Educ Nurs* 28(3):135-139, 1997.

Maloni JA, Ponder MB: Fathers' experience of their partners' antepartum bed rest, *Image: J Nurs Schol* 29:183-188, 1997.

McGown A, Whitbread J: Out of control! The most effective way to help the binge-eating patient, *J Psychosoc Nurs* 34:30-37, 1996.

Mohr WK: Outcomes of corporate greed, *Image: J Nurs Schol* 29:39-45, 1997.

Riordan J, Washburn J: Comparison of baccalaureate student lifestyle health behaviors entering and completing the nursing program, *J Nurs Educ* 36:262-265, 1997.

Sherman DW: Nurses' willingness to care for AIDS patients and spirituality, social support, and death anxiety, *Image: J Nurs Schol* 28:205-213, 1996.

Simpson G, Kenrick M: Nurses' attitudes toward computerization in clinical practice in a British General Hospital, *Computer Nurs* 15:37-32, 1997.

Ward SE, Berry PE, Misiewicz H: Concerns about analgesics among patients and family caregivers in a hospice setting, *Res Nurs Health* 19:205-211, 1996.

Qualitative Approaches to Research

9

Sharon A. Denham

Introduction

 Qualitative research continues to gain recognition as a sound method for investigating the complex human phenomena less easily explored using quantitative methods. Empirical studies are essential for investigating particular variables, but are less helpful in understanding human responses and life experiences. Nurse researchers and investigators from other disciplines are discovering the increased value of findings obtained through qualitative studies. Nurses can be better prepared to critique the appropriateness of a research design and identify the usefulness of the study findings when the differences between quantitative and qualitative research designs are understood.

Learning Outcomes

On completion of this chapter, the student should be able to do the following:
- Distinguish the characteristics of qualitative research from those of quantitative research.
- Recognize the uses of qualitative research.
- Identify the qualitative approaches of phenomenological, grounded theory, ethnographic, and historical methods.
- Evaluate a qualitative research report using critiquing criteria.

Activity 1

The reasons for selecting a qualitative design rather than a quantitative one are based upon the research question and the purpose of the study. Recognition of the differences of the characteristics of qualitative research from quantitative research enable the nurse to better interpret the research report findings and identify ways they might be applied.

1. Complete the following statements related to qualitative research characteristics.

   a. Qualitative research combines the _____ and _____ natures of nursing to better understand the human experience.

   b. Qualitative research is used to study human experience and life context in _____.

   c. Life context is the matrix of human-human-environment relationships that emerge through _____.

   d. Qualitative researchers study the _____ of individuals as they carry on their usual activities of daily life, which might occur at home, work, or school.

   e. The number of participants or subjects in a qualitative study is usually _____ than the number in a quantitative study.

   f. Quantitative research studies strive to eliminate extraneous variables, and qualitative studies are intended to explore _____ in order to better understand the participant experience.

   g. The choice to use either quantitative or qualitative methods is guided by the _____.

2. Match the following terms with the appropriate definitions:

A. Theoretical sampling
B. Emic
C. Etic
D. Data saturation
E. Secondary sources

F. Bracketed
G. Case study method
H. Grounded theory method
I. Domains
J. Key informants

a. _____ Information becomes repetitive

b. _____ Select experiences to test ideas

c. _____ Outsider's view

d. _____ Identify personal biases about phenomenon

e. _____ Insider's view

f. _____ Symbolic categories

g. _____ Individuals willing to teach investigator about the phenomenon

h. _____ In-depth description of phenomenon

i. _____ Provide another perspective of phenomenon

j. _____ Inductive approach to develop theory about social processes

3. Four qualitative research methods are discussed in the text in relationship to five basic elements of research. Under each research element, briefly describe a key aspect of this element in relationship to each of the four qualitative methods.

a. Element 1: Identifying the phenomenon

1. Phenomenology

2. Grounded theory

3. Ethnography

4. Historical

b. Element 2: Structuring the study

   1. Phenomenology

   2. Grounded theory

   3. Ethnography

   4. Historical

c. Element 3: Gathering the data

   1. Phenomenology

   2. Grounded theory

   3. Ethnography

   4. Historical

d. Element 4: Analyzing the data

   1. Phenomenology

   2. Grounded theory

   3. Ethnography

   4. Historical

e. Element 5: Describing the findings

   1. Phenomenology

   2. Grounded theory

   3. Ethnography

   4. Historical

4. Briefly describe a research topic that interests you, identify the qualitative approach you would choose to study this interest, and explain why.

Check your answers with those in Appendix A, Chapter 9

Activity 2

The literature review provides a background for understanding a research problem. All qualitative research methods do not include literature reviews, but the study entitled *Healing of Adult Male Survivors of Childhood Sexual Abuse* (1996) by Drauker and Petrovic did (Appendix B).

1. Read the literature review at the beginning of this study report and answer the following questions:

   a. What is the main theme of the literature review?

   b. Explain two ways this literature review could be applied to nursing practice.

   c. After reading this literature review, identify another topic area that the researchers might have included that would give you additional information for better understanding the problem of male abuse.

Check your answers with those in Appendix A, Chapter 9.

Activity 3

The theoretical underpinnings of qualitative research often make the findings directly applicable to nursing practice. Read the discussion and conclusion section of the Draucker and Petrovic (1996) report and answer the following questions.

1. The researchers identified the image of a dungeon as the way male abuse victims thought about the victimization they experienced. Read the ways the researchers used their data to describe the themes of living in the dungeon, breaking free, living free, and freeing those left behind, and answer the following items.

   a. True   False   Living in the dungeon was described by men as being confined, trapped, and silenced.

   b. True   False   Participants rarely identified a discrete or intense incident that began their healing.

   c. True   False   Feeling alive was described as awakening of senses and breaking out of the dungeon.

   d. True   False   The majority of males who experienced their own sense of freedom desired to free those still being oppressed or victimized.

   e. True   False   Most men believed their on-going healing would be a life-long effort.

   f. True   False   The findings of the study add to the literature by describing the healing process of male abuse victims as going from captivity to freedom.

   g. True   False   These study findings can easily be generalized to all male survivors.

   h. True   False   Attending to client's descriptions of personal abuse experiences can aid the understanding male victim's unique characteristics.

2. Qualitative research has many uses for nursing practice. After reading Drauker's and Petrovic's (1996) report, list ways that this research might be applied to nursing practice.

3. Research studies are infrequently replicated, but could provide greater understanding about the findings and might increase the useability of the findings. Explain where and how you might replicate this study with another population.

4. One finding from this study is the need for male abuse victims to have an opportunity to tell their stories of victimization. Give an example of how you might apply this knowledge to your present nursing practice.

Check your answers with those in Appendix A, Chapter 9.

Activity 4

Four qualitative methods of research are the phenomenological, grounded theory, ethnographic, and historical methods.

1. For each characteristic listed below, indicate which method of qualitative research it describes. Use the abbreviations from the key provided.

    Key: A = Phenomenological   C = Ethnographic
           B = Grounded theory   D = Historical

    a. _____   Uses primary and secondary sources.

    b. _____   Uses "emic" and "etic" views of subjects' worlds.

    c. _____   Research questions are action or change oriented.

    d. _____   Central meanings arise from subjects' descriptions of lived experience.

    e. _____   Truth is a lived experience.

    f. _____   Uses theoretical sampling to analyze data.

g. _____ Discovers "domains" to analyze data.

h. _____ Provides insight on the past and serves as a guide to the present and future.

i. _____ Establishes fact, probability, or possibility.

j. _____ States individuals' history is a dimension of the present.

k. _____ Attempts to discover underlying social forces that shape human behavior.

l. _____ Interviews "key informants."

m. _____ Presents data as a synthesized chronicle.

n. _____ Focuses on describing cultural groups.

o. _____ Establishes reliability through external and internal criticism.

p. _____ Researcher "brackets" personal bias or perspective.

q. _____ Subjects are currently experiencing a circumstance.

r. _____ Collects remembered information from subjects.

s. _____ Involves "field work."

t. _____ Describes events from the past.

u. _____ May use photographs to describe current behavioral practices.

v. _____ Uses symbolic interaction as a theoretical base.

w. _____ Uses an inductive approach to understanding basic social processes.

2. Review the research report *Healing of Adult Male Survivors of Childhood Sexual Abuse* by Draucker and Petrovic (1996) (Appendix B) and complete the following multiple choice items.

   a. What was the qualitative method used in the research study?

   (1) Phenomeological

   (2) Grounded theory

(3) Ethnography

(4) Historical

b. What social process was studied in this research?

(1) Childhood sexual abuse

(2) Victimization of men

(3) Male survivors of childhood sexual abuse

(4) Sexually abused males

c. What methods were used for data collection?

(1) Formal and unstructured interviews

(2) Observation

(3) Interviews and observation

(4) Participant observation

d. What were the methods for data analysis?

(1) Theoretical sampling

(2) Synthesis of essences

(3) Constant comparative method

(4) Both (1) and (3)

e. What were sample size and selection based upon?

(1) Data saturation and personal experience of the phenomenon

(2) Random selection

(3) Convenience sampling

(4) Advisement of key informants

3. Based on the four methods of qualitative research described in the text, answer the following:

   a.   Select the qualitative method you found the most interesting:

   b.   Explain the things you find especially appealing about this method:

   c.   List three subject areas this method might be helpful in developing nursing knowledge:

       (1)

       (2)

       (3)

   d.   Choose one of these subject areas and identify the research question to be studied:

   e.   Describe the data collection methods you would use for this study:

   f.   Identify the characteristics of the study subjects, where you will locate them, how many subjects you might include and why:

   g.   Briefly explain an important aspect of data analysis using this qualitative method:

   h.   Describe how you might use the knowledge gained from this study in nursing practice:

Check your answers with those in Appendix A, Chapter 9.

Posttest

1. True   False   Qualitative research focuses on the whole of human experiences in naturalistic settings.

2. True   False   External criticism in historical research refers to the authenticity of data sources.

3. True   False   In qualitative research one would expect the number of subjects participating to be as large as those usually found in quantitative studies.

4. True   False   The researcher is viewed as the major instrument for data collection.

5. True   False   Qualitative studies strive to eliminate extraneous variables.

6. To what does the term "saturation" in qualitative research refer?
   a.   Data repetition
   b.   Subject exhaustion
   c.   Researcher exhaustion
   d.   Sample size

7. In qualitative research, data are often collected by which of the following?
   a.   Questionnaires sent out to subjects
   b.   Observation of subjects in naturalistic settings
   c.   Interviews
   d.   All are correct

8. The qualitative method that uses symbolic interaction as the theoretical base for research is known as which of the following?
   a.   Phenomenology
   b.   Grounded theory
   c.   Ethnography
   d.   Historical method

9. What is the qualitative method that attempts to construct the meaning of the lived experience of human phenomena?
   a.   Phenomenology
   b.   Grounded theory
   c.   Ethnography
   d.   Historical method

10. What is the qualitative research method most appropriate for answering the question: "What changes in nursing practice occurred after the Viet Nam War?"
   a. Phenomenology
   b. Grounded theory
   c. Ethnography
   d. Historical method

11. What qualitative research method would be most appropriate for studying the impact of culture on the health behaviors of urban Hispanic youth?
   a. Phenomenology
   b. Grounded theory
   c. Ethnography
   d. Historical method

12. Which data analysis process is not used with grounded theory methodology?
   a. Bracketing
   b. Axial coding
   c. Theoretical sampling
   d. Open coding

The answers to the posttest are in the *Instructor's Resource Manual.*
Please check with your instructor for these answers.

References

Denham SA: Combatting the monster of domestic violence, *Nurs Forum* 30(3):12-19, 1995.

Denham SA: *An ethnographic study of family health in Appalachian microsystems* (unpublished dissertation), Birmingham, AL, 1997, University of Alabama at Birmingham.

Draucker CB, Petrovic K: Healing of adult male survivors of childhood sexual abuse, *Image: J Nurs Schol* 28(4):325-330, 1996.

Sampling

10

Ann Marttinen Doordan

Introduction

Sampling consists of choosing the elements to be used in answering the research question. The ideal sampling strategy is one in which the elements truly represent the population while controlling for any source of bias. Reality modulates the ideal. Considerations of efficiency, practicality, ethics, and availability of subjects frequently alter the ideal sampling strategy for a given study.

Learning Outcomes

On completion of this chapter, the student should be able to do the following:
- Identify the advantages and disadvantages of the following sampling strategies:
    a. Convenience sampling
    b. Quota sampling
    c. Purposive sampling
    d. Simple random sampling
    e. Stratified random sampling
    f. Cluster sampling
    g Systematic sampling
- Distinguish between probability and nonprobability sampling strategies.
- Identify the sampling strategy used in study examples.
- Evaluate the congruence between the sample used and population of interest.
- Critique the sampling component of a study.

Activity 1

Identify the category of sampling for each of the following sampling strategies. Use the abbreviations from the key provided.

Key: P = Probability sampling
       N = Nonprobability sampling

1. _____   Simple random sampling

2. _____   Purposive sampling

3. _____   Cluster sampling

4. _____   Quota sampling

5. _____   Convenience sampling

6. _____   Systematic sampling

7. _____   Stratified random sampling

Check your answers with those in Appendix A, Chapter 10.

Activity 2

For each of the following examples of studies, identify the sampling strategy used from the following list. Write the letter that corresponds to the strategy in the space preceding the sampling description.

Check the glossary for definition of terms.

    a. Convenience sampling
    b. Quota sampling
    c. Purposive sampling
    d. Simple random sampling
    e. Stratified random sampling
    f. Cluster sampling
    g. Systematic sampling

1. _____   The sample for the study of critical thinking behavior of undergraduate baccalaureate nursing students consisted of students enrolled in junior and senior level courses in three schools of nursing. In each program, students were invited to participate until a total sample representing 10% of the junior level students and 10% of the senior level students was obtained.

2. _____   Every eighth person on the diabetic clinic patient roster was asked to participate in the study. A table of random numbers was used to select the beginning of the sampling within the first sampling interval.

3. _____   Using a table of random numbers, the sample consisting of 50 subjects was selected from the list of all mothers giving birth in the county during the first 6 months of the year.

4. _____   The sample was selected from residents of eight nursing homes in Arkansas and consisted of cognitively impaired persons with no physical impairments or other psychiatric illness. (Beck et al, 1997)

5. _____   To select the sample, 25 rehabilitation centers were randomly selected from the list of all rehabilitation centers in the United States. Ten nurses were randomly selected from each site for a final sample of 250 nurses.

6. _____   The sample consisted of 23 chronic pain patients participating in a multimodal pain rehabilitation program. (Vines et al, 1996)

7. _____   To study educational opportunities for nurses from various ethnic groups, a list of all nurses in the state of California was sorted by ethnicity. The sample consisted of 10% of the nurses in each ethnic group, selected according to a table of random numbers.

Check your answers with those in Appendix A, Chapter 10.

Activity 3

1. Refer to the study by Wikblad and Anderson, *A Comparison of Three Wound Dressings in Patients Undergoing Heart Surgery*, in Appendix A of your textbook.

    a.   Was the sample adequately described?

        Yes   No

    b.   Do the sample characteristics correspond to the larger population?

        Yes   No   Partially

    c.   Is this a probability or nonprobability sample?

    d.   Is the sample size appropriate?

        Yes   No   Unsure

2. List one advantage of using a convenience sample in this study.

3. List one disadvantage of using a convenience sample.

Check your answers with those in Appendix A, Chapter 10.

Activity 4

Using the critical thinking decision path (Figure 10-3) and Table 10-1 in the textbook, label the following statements true or false.

    1. _____   Nonprobability sampling is associated with less generalizability to the larger population.

    2. _____   Convenience sampling followed by random assignment into treatment groups increases generalizability.

    3. _____   Nonprobability sampling strategies are more time consuming than probability strategies.

4. _____ Random sampling has the greatest risk of bias and is moderately representative.

5. _____ The advantage of ease of sampling is associated with the greatest risk of bias and limited representativeness of the sample.

6. _____ Purposive sampling produces the least generalizable sample of the sampling strategies listed.

Check your answers with those in Appendix A, Chapter 10.

Activity 5

Review the study by Rudy et al, *Patient Outcomes for the Chronically Critically Ill: Special care Unit Versus Intensive Care Unit*, in Appendix C in the textbook. Using the critiquing criteria listed in Chapter 10, critique the sampling process used in this study.

1. Have the sample characteristics been completely described? (Explain your answer.)

2. Can the parameters of the study population be inferred from the description of the sample?

3. To what extent is the sample representative of the population as defined?

4. Are criteria for eligibility in the sample specifically identified?

5. Have sample delimitations been established? (Explain your answer.)

6. Would it be possible to replicate the study population? (Explain your answer.)

7. How was the sample selected? Is the method of sample selection appropriate?

8. What kind of bias, if any, is introduced by this method?

9. Is the sample size appropriate? How is it substantiated?

10. Are there indications that rights of subjects have been ensured? (Explain your answer.)

11. Does the researcher identify the limitations in generalizability of the findings from the sample to the population? Are they appropriate?

12. Does the researcher indicate how replication of the study with other samples would provide increased support for the findings?

Check your answers with those in Appendix A, Chapter 10.

Posttest

Complete the sentences below.

1. Sampling strategies are grouped into two categories: _____ sampling and _____ sampling.

2. _____ sampling is the use of the most readily accessible persons or objects as subjects in a study.

3. Advantages of _____ sampling are low bias and maximal representativeness, but the disadvantage is the labor in drawing a sample.

4. A(n) _____ can be used to select an unbiased sample or unbiased assignment of subjects to treatment groups.

5. A(n) _____ sample is one whose key characteristics closely approximate those of the population.

6. _____ criteria are used to select the sample from all possible units and _____ may be used to restrict the population to a homogeneous group of subjects.

7. Types of nonprobability sampling include _____ , _____ , and _____ sampling.

8. Successive random sampling of units that progress from large to small and meet sample eligibility criteria is known as _____ sampling.

9. In certain qualitative studies, subjects are added to the sample until _____ occurs (new data no longer emerge during data collection).

10. A statistical technique known as _____ may be used to determine sample size in quantitative studies.

The answers to the posttest are in the *Instructor's Resource Manual*.
Please check with your instructor for these answers.

References

Beck C et al: Improving dressing behavior in cognitively impaired nursing home residents, *Nurs Res* 46:126-131, 1997.

Rudy EB et al: Patient outcomes for the chronically critically ill: special care unit versus intensive care unit, *Nurs Res* 44:324-331, 1995.

Vines SW et al: Effects of a multimodal pain rehabilitation program: a pilot study, *Rehab Nurs* 21:25-30, 1996.

Wikblad K, Anderson B: A comparison of three wound dressings in patients undergoing heart surgery, *Nurs Res* 44:312-316, 1995.

Legal and Ethical Issues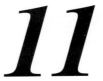

Mary Jo Gorney-Moreno

Introduction

Patient advocacy is one of the primary roles of a professional nurse. Nowhere is this more necessary than in the field of research. The nurse must be the client advocate, whether acting as the researcher, a participant in data gathering, or a provider of care for research subjects. A multitude of legal and ethical issues exist in research; nurses must be aware of, assess, and evaluate these issues. Nurses need to be knowledgeable about the purpose and functions of Institutional Review Boards and the federal regulations on which they are based.

Learning Outcomes

On completion of this chapter, the student should be able to do the following:
* Identify the essential elements of an informed consent form.
* Describe the Institutional Review Board's role in the research review process.
* Describe the nurse's role as patient advocate in research situations.
* Critique the ethical aspects of a research study.

Activity 1

Fill in the blanks with the correct term from the following list:

> Expedited Review
> Nursing Research Committee
> Justice
> Unethical Research Study
> Institutional Review Board

1. _____ reviews proposals for scientific merit and congruence with the institutional policies and missions.

2. The idea that human subjects should be treated fairly and no benefit to which a person is entitled should be denied is called _____.

3. A study of existing data that is of minimal risk may be a candidate for _____.

4. The US Public Health Service studied untreated syphilis on black sharecroppers in Tuskegee and withheld penicillin treatment even after penicillin was commonly available. This was considered a(n) _____.

5. _____ reviews research proposals to assure protection of the rights of human subjects.

Check your answers with those in Appendix A, Chapter 11.

Activity 2

List the *three* ethical principles relevant to the conduct of research involving human subjects.

1.

2.

3.

Check your answers with those in Appendix A, Chapter 11.

Activity 3

Review the articles in Appendices A-D of the text. For each article, describe how informed consent was obtained and how the author described obtaining permission from the Institutional Review Board (IRB).

1. Appendix A

2. Appendix B

3. Appendix C

4. Appendix D

Check your answers with those in Appendix A, Chapter 11.

Activity 4

1. Identify *at least four* groups of subjects who are vulnerable or have diminished autonomy.

   a.

   b.

   c.

   d.

2. Read the following study excerpts as if you are a nurse member of an IRB. Do you see any conditions that might require special circumstances? If yes, list them below.

   a. "The study examined the effect of individualized computerized testing system for baccalaureate nursing students enrolled in health assessment and obstetrics/women's health during a 3-year period. One hundred twenty-seven students participated in the study. The testing software, Pedagogue TM, was used to generate the computer test, and the students took all quizzes on-line. The mean score on computer tests in both courses were as good as, or better than previous scores on paper-pencil forms of the tests ($p<.05$)." (Bloom and Trice, 1997)

   Special circumstances?

   b. "Inner-city male adolescents in jail in New York City ($N = 427$) were interviewed to examine correlates of cocaine or crack use. Twenty-three percent had used cocaine or crack in the month before arrest and 32% reported lifetime use. Substantial rates of robbery, murder, other violent crime, weapons possession, and drug dealing were found. However, type of crime, including violent crime, was not related either to cocaine/crack use or to drug dealing. Current cocaine/crack users were more likely to use alcohol, marijuana, and intranasal heroin; to have multiple previous arrests; to be out of school; to be psychologically distressed; to have been sexually molested as a child; to have substance-abusing parents; and to have cocaine/crack-using friends. They were also more likely to have frequent sex with girls, to be gay or bisexual, and to engage in anal intercourse. The findings should be considered in developing more effective drug abuse prevention and treatment interventions, and HIV prevention and education for incarcerated at-risk adolescents." (Kang, Magura, and Shapiro, 1994)

   Special circumstances?

Check your answers with those in Appendix A, Chapter 11.

Activity 5

What is the composition of the IRB at your college or hospital? List the professions of the members.

Check your answers with those in Appendix A, Chapter 11.

Activity 6

In a discussion about the lack of agreement on what constitutes or does not constitute scientific misconduct, Hansen and Hansen (1995) have posed several questions to consider. The three questions that are most likely to be of concern to research consumers are listed below. For each, write your opinion below the question.

1. "Have you ever gotten a suggestion or idea for your research from a verbal comment (either in a lecture or directly to you) that you did not acknowledge in a later written report of the research?"

2. "Have you ever paraphrased a statement made by someone else without identifying the source?"

3. "Would you provide free access to your raw data to any researcher asking to use it after you have published your results?"

Check your answers with those in Appendix A, Chapter 11.

Activity 7

It is 1942, and you are the first doctorally prepared nurse at your hospital. You are approached by Sister Kinney to show the doctors that her treatment for spasms (i.e., paralysis of poliomyelitis) is the right way to treat patients. How would you respond to her? What would be your ethical concerns related to this research? (*Note:* A summary of Sister Kinney's methods and ideas follows.)

It may be helpful to read the fascinating article describing Kinney's life and ideas in *Image: Journal of Nursing Scholarship* First Quarter, p. 83-88, 1997.

By age 23, Elizabeth was an established bush nurse. She delivered babies and cared for the sick . . . in 1911, she encountered a young girl in constant pain, muscular pain that increased severely when touched. The child's legs were contracted in twisted positions, and her back and neck were misaligned. Confused by this condition, Nurse Elizabeth telegrammed Dr. McDonnell for advice. The return message stated: Infantile paralysis. No known treatment. Do the best you can with the symptoms presenting themselves. (Kinney and Ostenso, 1943; Morris, 1972; Oppewal, 1997)

Relying on keen observation, caring concern, and past knowledge from studying human anatomy, Elizabeth experimented to relieve the child's pain. She had never read or heard of a medical treatment for infantile paralysis, or poliomyelitis, as it was later called. Fearful that contractures and deformities would permanently result unless the child's muscles relaxed, she tried applying heated salt placed in a bag and a linseed meal poultice. Both were too heavy. However, the child did respond to heat from a wool blanket torn into strips then placed in boiling water and wrung dry. Upon awakening from a relaxed sleep, the child said, "I want them rags that wells my legs!" (Kinney and Ostenso, 1943)

A year elapsed before Elizabeth discussed this first, and five other cases with Dr. McDonnell. He was surprised to learn that none of her patients developed deformities. The orthodox medical treatment at that time was to immobilize the affected limbs during the painful period. Deformity resulted when the healthy muscle in a muscle pair pulled the affected muscle out of shape. Unfortunately, many polio victims treated with immobilization sustained some type of crippling. Elizabeth explained that she successfully treated spasms with moist heat . . . (Kinney and Ostenso, 1943)

Although many patients who were treated with the Kenny method achieved relief and did not develop deformities, her methods were not endorsed by the medical community in Australia. Instead, she was ridiculed by the medical community and accused of being politically motivated. After the death of her main supporter, Dr. McDonnell, who had stated: "She has knocked our theories into a cocked hat, but her treatment works, and that's all that counts"; she decided to bring her ideas to the United States. (Kinney and Ostenso, 1943)

Following her arrival in America, Kinney again received little support from the medical community. Even though Sister Kinney understood the importance of obtaining medical sanction, she recognized the revolutionary nature of her method . . . To avoid being labeled a quack Sister Kenny realized that her method had to receive scientific validation. (Levine, 1954). Yet, she vacillated between a mission of research and one of instruction. For example, she stated, "I came to America to teach my method—not to enter a research experiment." (Potter, 1941)

Kinney realized that American physicians wanted systematic proof that her empirically demonstrated method worked. But performing a valid experiment on the Kinney method of immobilization raised ethical problems. No parents would allow their children to receive a treatment that was not the most effective that medicine could offer. (Kinney and Ostenso, 1943; Potter, 1941)

1. What is your response to her?

2. What are the major ethical issues involved in the design of this study?

3. How would you design a research study to determine the most effective treatment for spasms in poliomyelitis?

Check your answers with those in Appendix A, Chapter 11.

Posttest

Fill in the blank with the correct term.

1. A researcher must receive some form of IRB approval (before; after) _____ beginning to conduct research involving humans.

2. If you question whether a researcher has permission to conduct a study in your hospital, you would want to see a document demonstrating approval from which group(s)?

3. Should a researcher list all the possible risks and benefits of participating in a research study? Circle one   Yes   No

4. If you agreed to collect data for a researcher who had not asked the patient's permission to participate in the research study, you would be violating the patient's right to:

The answers to the posttest are in the *Instructor's Resource Manual*.
Please check with your instructor for these answers.

References

Bloom K, Trice L: The efficacy of individualized computerized testing in nursing education, *Computer Nurs* 15:82-88, 1997.

Draucker B, Petrovic K: Healing of adult male survivors of childhood sexual abuse, *Image: J Nurs Schol* 28:325-330, 1996.

Hansen BC, Hansen KD: Academic and scientific misconduct: issues for nursing educators, *J Prof Nurs* 11(1):31-39, 1995.

Kang SY, Magura S, Shapiro JL: Correlates of cocaine/crack use among inner-city incarcerated adolescents, *Am J Drug Alcohol Abuse* 20:413-429, 1994.

Oppewal SR: Sister Elizabeth Kinney, an Australian nurse, and treatment of poliomyelitis victims, *Image: J Nurs Schol* 29:83-87, 1997.

Rempusheski VE, Wolfe BE, Dow KH, Fish LC: Peer review by nursing research committees in hospitals, *Image: J Nurs Schol* 28:51-53, 1996.

Rudy EB et al: Patient outcomes for the chronically critically ill: special care unit versus intensive care unit, *Nurs Res* 44:324-331, 1995.

Ward SE, Berry PE, Misiewicz H: Concerns about analgesics among patients and family caregivers in a hospice setting, *Res Nurs Health* 19:205-211, 1996.

Wikblad K, Anderson B: A comparison of three wound dressings in patients undergoing heart surgery, *Nurs Res* 44:312-316, 1995.

Data Collection Methods *12*

Martha Rock

Introduction

Observe, probe
Details unfold
Let nature's secrets
Be stammeringly retold.
—Goethe

The focus of this chapter is basic information about data collection. As a consumer of research the reader needs the skills to evaluate and critique data collection methods in published research studies. In order to achieve these skills it is helpful to have an appreciation of the process or the critical thinking "journey" the researcher has taken to be ready to collect the data. Each of the preceding chapters represented important preliminary steps in the research planning and designing phases prior to data collection. Although most researchers are eager to begin data collection, the planning for data collection is very important. The planning includes identifying and prioritizing data needs, developing or selecting appropriate data collection tools, and selecting and training data collection personnel before proceeding with actual collection of data.

The five types of data collection methods differ in their basic approach and the strengths and weaknesses of their characteristics. Readers should be prepared to ask questions about the appropriateness of the measures chosen by the researcher to gather data about the variable of concern. This includes determining the objectivity, consistency, quantifiability, observer intervention, and/or obtrusiveness of the chosen data collection method.

Learning Outcomes

On completion of this chapter, the reader should be able to do the following:
- Describe the five types of data collection methods used in nursing research.
- Describe the advantages and disadvantages of selected data collection methods.
- Match types of variables to the most appropriate data collection method.
- Critique data collection components of the methodology of specific studies.
- Evaluate the applicability of published research studies based upon a critique of their data collection method.
- Discuss the role of data collection in the overall research process.

Activity 1

Review each of the articles referenced below; be especially thorough in reading the sections that relate to data collection methods. Answer the questions in relation to what you understand from the article. For some questions, there may be more than one answer.

Study 1

Wikblad K, Anderson B: A comparison of three wound dressings in patients undergoing heart surgery, *Nurs Res* 44(5):312-316, 1995. (Appendix A of the text)

1. Which data collection method is used in this research study?
    a. A physiological measure
    b. An observational measure
    c. An interview measure
    d. A questionnaire measure
    e. Records or available data

2. Rationale for appropriateness of method:

3. Interrater reliability is a very important issue. What steps were implemented to assure this consistency in each of the measurement areas in the study?

    a. Nurses' protocol

       Level of agreement

    b. Photographic protocol

       Level of agreement

c. Public health nurses' protocol

Level of agreement

Study 2

Draucker CB, Petrovic K: Healing of adult male survivors of childhood sexual abuse, *Image: J Nurs Schol* 28(4):325-330, 1996. (Appendix B of the text)

1. Which data collection method is used in this research study?
   a. A physiological measure
   b. An observational measure
   c. An interview measure
   d. A questionnaire
   e. Records or available data

2. In grounded theory studies the concepts emerge from the data; therefore the questions should be _____.
   a. Open-ended
   b. Close-ended
   c. Tape-recorded
   d. Time-limited

3. What was the rationale for some researcher contacts being face-to-face and some being telephone contacts?

4. Rationale for appropriateness of data collection method:

Study 3

Rudy EB et al: Patient outcomes for the chronically critically ill: special care unit versus intensive care unit, *Nurs Res* 44(8):324-332, 1995. (Appendix C of the text)

1. What data collection method is used in this research study?
   a. A physiological measure
   b. An observational measure
   c. An interview measure
   d. A questionnaire
   e. Records or available data

2. As you review this study, it is evident that several changes had to be made after the study began. What could have prevented these problems from occurring in this study?
   a. Better screening of clients
   b. Better training of evaluators
   c. Different data collection method
   d. Pilot study

3. As you critique this study, give the rationale for the appropriateness of the data collection method.

4. Describe the way consistency was maintained in this study.

Study 4

Ward SE, Berry PE, Misiewicz H: Concerns about analgesics among patients and family caregivers in a hospice setting, *Res Nurs Health* 19:205-211, 1996. (Appendix D of the text)

1. What data collection method is used in this research study?
   a. A physiological measure
   b. An observational measure
   c. An interview measure
   d. A questionnaire
   e. Records or available data

2. Two variables the researchers studied were *hesitancy to report pain* and *hesitancy to use analgesics*.
   a. Open-ended questions were asked to elicit this information.
   b. Close-ended questions were asked to elicit this information.

3. Write a critiquing statement that includes three areas of evaluation for this study.

Check your answers with those in Appendix A, Chapter 12.

Activity 2

Using the content of Chapter 12 in the text, have fun with the *Word Search Exercise*. Answer the questions below and find the word in the puzzle.

1. Baccalaureate prepared nurses are _____ of research.
2. _____ are those methods that use technical instruments to collect data about patients' physical, chemical, microbiological, or anatomical status.
3. _____ is the distortion of data as a result of the observer's presence.
4. _____ are best used when a large response rate and an unbiased sample are important.
5. _____ data collection method is subject to problems of availability, authenticity, and accuracy.
6. _____ measurements are especially useful when there are finite number of questions to be asked and the questions are clear and specific.
7. Essential in the critique of data collection methods is the emphasis on the appropriateness, _____, and _____ of the method employed.
8. _____ raises ethical questions (especially informed consent issues); therefore, it is not used much in nursing.
9. _____ _____ is the consistency of observations between two or more observers.
10. _____ is the process of translating the concepts/variables into measurable phenomena.
11. _____ is a format that uses close-ended items, and there are a fixed number of alternative responses.
12. _____ is the method for objective, systematic, and quantitative description of communications and documentary evidence.
13. This exercise is supposed to be _____!

```
D E L I V E R S T A T I S T C S Y E S P A S
S S A C A B I N E T F O R K A Z O S P E I O
I A W O P E R A T I O N A L I Z A T I O N B
G T S N O R N E V E R B Y D N E A U X B T J
N S Y S T E M A T I C A J H T B S D V S E E
I F L I K E R T V E S O B E R R O Y A E R C
F A K S C A L E S N O V N O C A A U L R R T
H C U T A C R A T I M A P V E T P U I V A I
Y T B E B H I R T E M A H V W K I C D A T V
P C O N T E N T A N A L Y S I S P V O T E I
R O Y C B K D S I S R T S A D V A N E I R T
E R E Y O D U G K A T P I B I O I O G O R Y
A V S I B R Q U E S T I O N N A I R E N E C
C I A R E S E A R C H L L R E A C E S O L O
T O B M E X C E L A E O O D A T A C O V I N
I U E A E V A L I D S T G N O S T O O E A S
V N Y E S S I N T E R V I E W S A R F R B U
I H A P P I E N E S S P C A T A G D U N I M
T X C I T E D E L P H I A T O T P S N V L E
Y A B L E A C O N C E A L M E N T O O T T R
A I K E V A L I K E I I A B C O N S U M Y S
```

Check your answers with those in Appendix A, Chapter 12.

Activity 3

You are reviewing a study and concealment is necessary; in other words, there is no other way to collect the data and the data collected are unlikely to have negative consequences for the subject.

1. Give a specific example of what kind of study this might be.

2. How would you obtain subjects' consent?

3. What is this process called?

Check your answers with those in Appendix A, Chapter 12.

Activity 4

You are asked to participate in discussions about impending research in your community. The purpose of the study is to identify the health status, beliefs, practices, preventive services currently known and used and accessibility/availability of health service needs for the residents of your rural community.

Take me on your critical thinking journey . . . .
Describe what you would consider in the selection of a data collection method. Review each method and discuss the pros and cons for choosing a specific data collection method. State your rationale for your final selection. What would be your thinking about instruments and types?

Check your answers with those in Appendix A, Chapter 12.

Activity 5

Using the content of Chapter 12 in the textbook, circle the correct response for each question. Some questions will have more than one answer.

1. What is a primary advantage of physiological measures?
    a. The measuring tool never affects the phenomena that are being measured
    b. One of the easiest types of methods to implement
    c. The unlikelihood that study participants/subjects can distort the physiological information
    d. Their objectivity, sensitivity, and precision
    e. All of the above

2. Self-report measures are usually more useful than observation measures in obtaining information about which of the following?
   a. Socially unacceptable or private behaviors
   b. Complex research situations when it is difficult to separate processes and interactions
   c. When the researcher is interested in character traits
   d. All of the above

3. Which of the following would be considered disadvantages of using observational data collection methods?
   a. Individual bias may interfere with the data collection
   b. Ethical concerns may be increasingly significant to researchers using observational data collection methods
   c. Individual judgments and values influence the perceptions of the observers
   d. All of the above

4. In nursing research, when might questionnaires be used as an appropriate method for data collection?
   a. Whenever expense is a concern for the researcher
   b. When a researcher is interested in obtaining information directly from the subjects
   c. When the researcher needs to collect data from a large group of subjects that are not easily accessible
   d. When accuracy is of the utmost importance to the researcher

5. Which of the following would be considered advantages of using existing records or available data to answer a research question?
   a. The use of available data reduces the risk of researcher bias in data collection
   b. Time involvement in the research study can be reduced by the use of available records or data
   c. Consistent collection of information over periods of time allows the researcher to study trends
   d. All of the above

Check your answers with those in Appendix A, Chapter 12.

Posttest

Read each question thoroughly and then circle the correct answer. For some questions more than one answer may be correct.

1. What is the process of translating concepts that are of interest to the researcher into observable and measurable phenomena?
   a. Objectivism
   b. Systematization
   c. Subjectivism
   d. Operationalization

2. Answering research questions pertaining to psychosocial variables can best be answered by using which data gathering technique(s)?
   a. Observation
   b. Interviews
   c. Questionnaires
   d. All of the above

3. What is collection of data from each subject in the same or in a similar manner known as?
   a. Repetition
   b. Dualism
   c. Consistency
   d. Recidivism

4. What is consistency of observations between two or more observers known as?
   a. Intrarater reliability
   b. Interrater reliability
   c. Consistency reliability
   d. Repetitive reliability

5. Physiological and biological measurement might be used by nurse researchers when studying which of these variables?
   a. A comparison of student nurses' ACT scores and their GPAs
   b. Hypertensive clients' responses to a stress test
   c. Children's dietary patterns
   d. The degree of pain relief achieved following guided imagery

6. Scientific observations should fulfill which of the following conditions?
   a. Observations are consistent with the study objectives
   b. Observations are standardized and systematically recorded
   c. Observations are checked and controlled
   d. All of the above

7. In a research study, a participant observer spent regularly scheduled hours in a homeless shelter and occasionally stayed overnight. The people staying in the home were told that this person was conducting a research study. The researcher freely engaged in conversation and openly observed the homeless. What is the observational role of the researcher?
   a. Concealment without intervention
   b. Concealment with intervention
   c. No concealment without intervention
   d. No concealment with intervention

8. In unstructured observation, which of the following might occur?
   a. Extensive field notes are recorded
   b. Subjects are informed what behaviors are being observed
   c. The researcher frequently records interesting anecdotes
   d. All of the above

9. Which of the following is not consistent with a Likert scale?
   a. It contains close-ended items
   b. It contains open-ended items
   c. It contains lists of statements
   d. Items are evaluated on the amount of agreement

10. Although it is acceptable to use multiple instruments within a research study, the study is more acceptable if only one method is used for the data collection.
    a. True
    b. False

11. Social desirability is seldom a concern for researchers when the data collection method used in the study is interviews.
    a. True
    b. False

12. A researcher desires to use a questionnaire in a study but cannot find one that will gather the information desired about a particular variable. The decision is made to develop a new instrument. Which of the following should the researcher do?
    a. Define the construct, formulate the items, and assess the items for content validity
    b. Develop instructions for users and pilot the instrument
    c. Estimate reliability and validity
    d. All of the above

13. The researcher who invests significant amounts of time in the development of an instrument has a professional responsibility to publish the results.
    a. True
    b. False

14. In order to evaluate the adequacy of various data collection methods, which of the following should be observed in the written research report?
    a. Clear identification of the rationale for selecting a physiological measure
    b. The problems of bias and reactivity are addressed with observational measures
    c. There is a clear explanation of how interviews were conducted and how interviewers were trained
    d. All of the above

15. In conducting a research study, the researcher has a responsibility to ensure that all study subjects received the same information and data was collected from all participants in the same manner.
    a. True
    b. False

The answers to the posttest are in the *Instructor's Resource Manual*.
Please check with your instructor for these answers.

Reliability and Validity 13

Ann Marttinen Doordan

Introduction

The reliability and validity of the data collection instruments must be sound in order to have any confidence in the results. Any consumer of research must be able to critique the reliability and validity of instruments used in a research study. During the conduct of research, the possibility of systematic and random error must be kept to a minimum in order to believe the results of the study.

Learning Outcomes

On completion of this chapter, the student should be able to do the following:
*   Discuss reliability and validity as they relate to data collection instruments.
*   Compare content, criterion, and construct validity in the choice of instruments used in research.
*   Compare stability, homogeneity, and equivalence in determining reliability.
*   Critique the reliability and validity reported in research studies.

Activity 1

Either random error (R) or systematic error (S) may occur in a research study. For each of the following examples, identify the type of measurement error and how the error might be corrected.

1. _____ The scale used to obtain daily weights was inaccurate by 3 pounds less than actual weight.
   Correction:

2. _____ Students chose the socially acceptable responses on an instrument to assess attitudes toward AIDS patients.
   Correction:

3. _____ Confusion existed among the evaluators on how to score the wound healing.
   Correction:

4. _____ The subjects were nervous about taking the psychological tests.
   Correction:

Check your answers with those in Appendix A, Chapter 13.

Activity 2

Validity is the concern whether the measurement tools are actually measuring what they are supposed to measure. Select a term or method from the list that best completes the following sentences.

Consult the glossary for assistance with definition of terms.

Concurrent validity
Content validity
Contrasted groups
Construct validity
Convergent
Criterion validity
Divergent
Face validity
Factor analysis
Hypothesis testing
Multitrait-multimethod approach
Predictive validity
Rating from a panel of experts

1. The three major kinds of validity are _____, _____, and
   _____.

2. A researcher used _____ to establish content validity of a new rating scale
   for maternal attachment.

3. _____ validity was assessed by correlating scores of the Learned Helplessness Scale with the Beck Hopelessness Scale and Rosenberg Self-Esteem Scale (Flynn,
   1997).

4. In the same study, Flynn (1997) used Radloff's Center for Epidemiologic Studies Depression Scale (CES-D). _____ validity was found through factor analyses that consistently supported the four theoretical categories of the instrument.

5. _____ is the use of a variety of measurement strategies to assess convergent and divergent validity.

6. _____ validity is an intuitive, preliminary type of instrument evaluation.

7. Construct validity, an assessment of the theory underlying the instrument, can be measured in several ways. List two of these: _____ and _____.

8. A researcher wants to establish construct validity of an instrument to measure social support using two other instruments. _____ validity was expected with the instrument that measured a construct similar to coping. _____ validity was expected with the instrument that measured a construct opposite to coping.

Check your answers with those in Appendix A, Chapter 13.

Activity 3

An instrument is considered reliable if it is accurate and consistent. If the concept being studied is stable, the same results should occur when measurement is repeated.

1. Three concepts related to reliability include _____ , _____ , and _____ .

2. Give an example of each of the two types of tests for stability.

3. In what instance would it be better to use an alternate form rather than a test-retest measure for stability?

4. Homogeneity is a measure of internal consistency. All items on the instrument should be complementary and measure the same characteristic or concepts. For each of the following examples, identify which of the following tests for homogeneity is described:
   (1) Item-total correlations
   (2) Split-half reliability
   (3) Kuder-Richardson (KR-20) coefficient
   (4) Cronbach's alpha

   a. _____ The odd items of the test had a high correlation with the even numbers of the test.
   b. _____ Each item on the test using a 5-point Likert scale had a moderate correlation with every other item on the test.
   c. _____ Each item on the test ranged in correlation from 0.62 to 0.89 with the total.
   d. _____ Each item on the true-false test had a moderate correlation with every other item on the test.

5. In the Rudy et al study in Appendix C, four ICU nurses were trained in the use of a scoring system. The scores for the nurses evaluating the same patients were compared and reported as a correlation coefficient. This is known as _____ reliability.

Check your answers with those in Appendix A, Chapter 13.

Activity 4

In this activity we will use the critiquing criteria listed in Chapter 13 to evaluate instruments used in the 1995 study by Rudy et al: *Patient Outcomes for the Chronically Critically Ill: Special Care Unit versus Intensive Care Unit* found in Appendix C of the text.
Refer to the section discussing the LaMonica-Oberst Patient Satisfaction Scale to answer the following questions.

1. The range of the original internal consistency (homogeneity/reliability) of the three subscales was 0.80 to 0.90. Is this acceptable?
   Yes   No

2. The alpha coefficient for the revised scale is 0.92. Is this adequate for reliability?
   Yes   No

3. How was the validity of the instrument evaluated? _____

4. Is the validity adequate?
   Yes   No

5. Did the researchers recalculate the validity and reliability of the revised instrument?
   Yes   No

6. Are the strengths and weaknesses of the reliability and validity of this instrument presented?
   Yes   No

Use the section on the Life-Threatening Complication Index (LTCI) for the next question.

7. How did the researchers maintain high interrater reliability for the scoring of this instrument?

Check your answers with those in Appendix A, Chapter 13.

Posttest

Using the following terms, complete the sentences for the type of validity or reliability discussed. Terms may be used more than one time.

Content validity	Test-retest reliability
Factor analysis	Cronbach's alpha
Convergent validity	Alternate or parallel form
Divergent validity	Interrater reliability

1. In tests for reliability the self-efficacy scale had a(n) _____ of 0.88, demonstrating internal consistency for the new measure.

2. The ABC social support scale demonstrated _____ validity with correlation of 0.84 with the XYZ interpersonal relationships scale.

3. _____ validity was supported with a correlation of 0.42 between the ABC social support scale and the QRS loneliness scale.

4. The investigator established _____ validity through evaluation of the cardiac recovery scale by a panel of cardiac clinical nurse specialists. All items were rated 0 to 5 for importance to recovery and only items scoring above an average of 3 were kept in the final scale.

5. The results of the _____ were that all the items clustered around three factors, lending support to the notion that there are three dimensions of coping.

6. The observations were rated by three experts. The _____ reliability among the observers was 94%.

7. To assess _____ reliability, subjects completed the locus of control questionnaire at the beginning of the project and 2 weeks later. The correlation of 0.86 supports the stability of the concept.

8. Bennett et al (1996) developed an instrument: the Cardiac Event Threat Questionnaire (CTQ). They established _____ validity by reviewing the literature, reviewing concerns identified by patients recovering from a cardiac event, and had the items critiqued by a panel of experts.

9. The results of the CTQ that measured threat were highly correlated with the results of a test measuring negative emotions. This established _____ validity.

10. Bennett et al (1996) reported that internal consistency reliabilities of the five factors of the CTQ were computed with the _____ statistic.

The answers to the posttest are in the *Instructor's Resource Manual*.
Please check with your instructor for these answers.

References

Bennett SJ et al: Development of an instrument to measure threat related to cardiac events, *Nurs Res* 45:266-270, 1996.

Flynn L: The health practices of homeless women: a causal model, *Nurs Res* 46:72-77, 1997.

Rudy EB et al: Patient outcomes for the chronically critically ill: special care unit versus intensive care unit, *Nurs Res* 44:324-331, 1995.

Descriptive Data Analysis 14

Kathleen Rose-Grippa

Introduction

Measurement is critical to any study. The researcher begins to think about how to measure the variables while reading the literature and thinking through the theoretical rationale for the study. Formulating the operational definitions is often the first direct link to the concept of measurement. These operational definitions point to relevant data collection instruments that in turn point to data analysis strategies. Seldom does a researcher have the luxury of defining the variables exactly as desired leading to ideal data collection instrument(s) that perfectly match analytical strategies. Your task as a critical reader of research is to consider all of the steps taken by the researcher and then ask "Did the researcher use the descriptive statistical tools that provide the clearest possible summary of the data?"

Common places to look for descriptive statistics will be in the descriptions of the individuals who participated in the study and to describe general information about the sample. Some studies will rely on descriptive statistics as the major data analysis strategy, and other studies will use a combination of descriptive and inferential statistics. This chapter focuses on the use of descriptive statistics.

First, the exercises in this chapter will provide you with some practice in working with the concept of measurement. Second, you will have the opportunity to think through some of the decisions relevant to the use of descriptive statistics. Descriptive statistics are used to describe the information from samples. Most studies use descriptive statistics to describe the individuals who participated in the study. Some studies will rely on descriptive statistics as the major data analysis strategy and other studies will use a combination of descriptive and inferential statistics. This chapter focuses on the use of descriptive statistics.

LEARNING OBJECTIVES

On completion of this chapter, the student should be able to do the following:

- Distinguish among the four levels of measurement.
- Identify the level of measurement used in specified sets of data.
- Recognize the symbols associated with specific descriptive statistical tools.
- Interpret accurate measures of central tendency and measures of variation.
- Critically evaluate the use of descriptive statistics in specified studies.

Activity 1

Match the level of measurement found in Column B with the appropriate example(s) in Column A. The levels of measurement in Column B will be used more than once.

Column A   **Column B**

1. _____ Amount of emesis   a. Nominal

2. _____ Scores on the ACT, SAT, or the GRE   b. Ordinal

3. _____ Height or weight   c. Interval

4. _____ High, moderate, low level of social support   d. Ratio

5. _____ Satisfaction with nursing care

6. _____ Use or nonuse of contraception

7. _____ Amount of empathy

8. _____ Number of feet or meters walked

9. _____ Type A or Type B behavior

10. _____ Body temperature measured with Centigrade thermometer

Activity 2

1. Read the following excerpts from specific studies. Identify the variable (or variables) and indicate what level of measurement would apply.
   You may find the Critical Thinking Decision Path from Chapter 14 of the textbook to be very helpful in answering these questions.

   a. "Mood state was defined as the client's full range of feelings about participation in the drug trial and was measured using the Bipolar Form of the Profile of Mood States" (Lorr, McNair, 1984, 1988). "The four-point Likert-type scale contained 72 items measuring mood over the previous week" (Wineman et al, 1996).

   Name of variable

   Level of measurement

b. "Perceived health status of the subjects was determined by asking them to choose one statement indicating their current state of physical health. Choices ranged from 1, indicating that "I think my present health is very good" to 5, indicating "I think my present health is very poor" (Johnson, 1996).

Name of variable

Level of measurement

c. "The Abuse Assessment Screen (AAS) was designed by the Nursing Research Consortium on Violence and Abuse . . . Abuse status on the AAS was determined by a yes' response to Question 2 ("Within the last year, have you been hit, slapped, kicked or otherwise physically hurt by someone?"), Question 3 ("Since you've been pregnant have you been hit, slapped, kicked, or otherwise physically hurt by someone?"), or Question 4 ("Within the last year, has anyone forced you to have sexual activities?")" (McFarlane, Parker and Soeken, 1996).

Name of variable

Level of measurement

d. "Diet diaries were kept for 3 days (2 weekdays and 1 weekend day). Each subject's dietary intake of carbohydrate, protein, and fat was used to calculate total calories and calories from each nutrient group . . . Diet diaries were analyzed using Food Processor software (ESHA Research, Salem, OR)" (Lipp, Deane, and Trimble, 1996).

Name of variable

Level of measurement

e. "Data were obtained from local health department records and a birth certificate data tape of the State of Illinois. Information gathered from the nursing and WIC records included . . . mother's age at delivery . . . trimester of initial PHN contact with client . . . infant birthweight . . ." (Baldwin and Chen, 1996).

Name of variable

Level of measurement

2. You have walked through the identification of the level of measurement based on information from the study about the variable. Now look at the report of the data used in Question 1 of this activity and decide if the appropriate descriptive statistic was used. Again, you may find the Critical Thinking Decision Path from Chapter 14 of the textbook useful.

Table 1. Means, Standard Deviations, and Ranges for Study Scales

Scales	Mean	Standard Deviation	Study Range	Possible Range
Mood state	40.7	36.65	-41 to 123	-197 to 233
Hopefulness	184.7	26.14	108 to 237	48 to 240
Illness uncertainty	77.3	10.07	57 to 106	27 to 135
Perceived stress	23.1	25.39	0 to 92	0 to 100
Coping effectiveness	159.3	77.20	0 to 326	0 to 360

N = 59.

Wineman NM et al: Relationships among illness uncertainty, stress, coping, and emotional well-being at entry into a clinical drug trial, Appl Nurs Res 9(2):53-60, 1996.

a. Review your answer to Question 1a and refer to Table 1.

What is the variable of interest in this table?

What part of Table 1 requires your attention?

b. Name the types of statistics used to describe the information about mood state.

c. Using the Critical Thinking Decision Path found in Chapter 14 of the textbook, what level of measurement is needed to use the statistics you named?

d. Does the level of measurement named in your answer to Question 2c match the level of measurement you indicated in your answer to Question 1a?
Yes   No

e. Once again you identified "abuse" or "abuse status" as the variable from the earlier excerpt from this study. Table 1 provides information about this variable and some other information. Are the appropriate descriptive statistics used to present these data? Explain your answer.

Table 2. Characteristics of Pregnant Women

	African American (n = 414)	Hispanic (n = 412)	White (n = 377)	Total (N = 1,203)
	Percent	Percent	Percent	Percent
Physical-Sexual Abuse				
Within last year	26.8	18.6	27.8	24.4
During pregnancy	18.3	13.1	16.7	16.0
Entered Prenatal Care at Third Trimester				
All women	12.8	8.0	8.8	9.9
Abused	19.3	13.1	10.4	14.5
Nonabused	10.1	6.5	8.1	8.2
Low-Birth-Weight (< 2,500 g) Deliveries	17.9	4.2	6.6	9.5

McFarlane J, Parker B, Soeken K: Abuse during pregnancy: associations with maternal health and infant birth weight, Nurs Res 45(1):37-42, 1996.

f. Refer to the data in Table 2. If you had only these data, what patterns would you expect to find discussed in the narrative portion of the study?

Table 3. Diet Diary*

	Mean	Range	SD
Total calories/d	3322	435-7753	1263
Total g of fat/d	132	17-334	58.3
% of total calories/d in fat	34	18-48	5.19
Total mg sodium/d	5369	840-9999	2189

*N = 78.

Lipp EJ, Deane D, Trimbe N: Cardiovascular disease risks in adolescent males, Appl Nurs Res 9(3):102-107, 1996.

g. Refer to your information in Question 1d. Are the data in Table 3 reported using the appropriate descriptive statistics for the level of measurement? Explain you answer.

h.   Write a narrative interpretation of the data in the first line of Table 3.

Check your answers with those in Appendix A, Chapter 14.

Activity 3

If you have taken a course in statistics, you are familiar with the statistical notation used to refer to specific types of descriptive statistics. This activity will serve as a quick review. For those of you who have not yet taken a statistics course, this exercise will provide enough information for you to recognize some of the statistical notations.

(*Note:* This is a *reverse* crossword puzzle, therefore, the puzzle is already completed. Your task is to identify the appropriate clue for each answer of the crossword puzzle.)

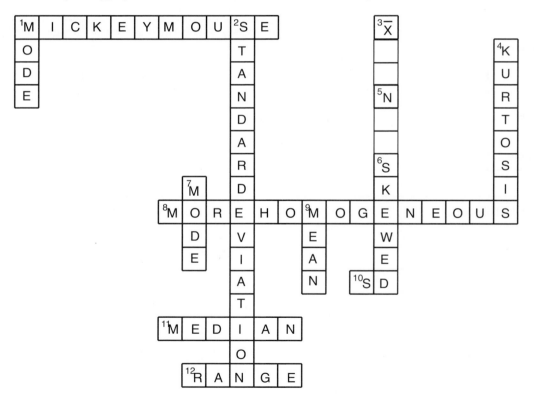

The Clues

- Measure of central tendency used with interval or ratio data.
- Abbreviation for the number of measures in a given data set (the measures may be individual people or some smaller piece of data like blood pressure readings).
- Measure of variation that shows the lowest and highest number in a data set.
- Can describe the height of a distribution.
- Old abbreviation for the mean.
- Marks the "score" where 50% of the scores are higher and 50% are lower.
- Describes a distribution characterized by a tail.
- Abbreviation for standard deviation.
- 68% of the values in a normal distribution fall between ±1 of this statistic.
- Goofy's best friend.
- Very unstable.
- The values that occur most frequently in a data set.
- Describes a set of data with a standard deviation of 3 when compared to a set of data with a standard deviation of 12.

Across	Down
1.	1.
3.	2.
5.	4.
8.	6.
10.	7.
11.	9.
12.	

Activity 4

You have now had some experience with matching variables, levels of measurement, and types of descriptive techniques. It is time to move to interpretation and critiquing of the use of descriptive statistics. A table from a research study is duplicated below. The Goodwin study was designed to describe the association among several measures of the marital relationship and the health of the wife with chronic fatigue and immune dysfunction syndrome (CFIDS). Study the information in Table 4 and answer the questions that follow.

Table 4. Means, Standard Deviations, and Paired t Tests for Husbands' and Wives' Scores

Scales	Husbands' M (SD)	Wives' M (SD)	n	t
Marital variables				
Marital adjustment	110.63 (18.13)	110.15 (17.74)	127	.36
Marital empathy				
Spouse ability	45.21 (14.44)	46.20 (15.68)	114	-.66
Self ability	32.66 (7.83)	33.58 (6.32)	115	-1.17
Marital support	52.66 (7.80)	53.22 (9.87)	130	-.71
Marital conflict	28.59 (8.43)	27.65 (9.50)	127	1.10
CFIDS symptoms				
Number of symptoms	42.97 (11.86)	46.73 (8.28)	128	-3.82***
Mean problem score	2.83 (0.69)	3.03 (0.58)	128	-3.40**
Total problem score	121.16 (44.16)	142.63 (39.30)	128	-6.80***

*p < .05. **p < .01. ***p < .001; 2 tailed
Note: CIFDS = chronic fatigue and immune dysfunction syndrome.
Goodwin SS: The marital relationship and health in women with chronic fatigue and immune dysfunction syndrome: views of wives and husbands, Nurs Res 46(3):138-146, 1997.

1. What is the highest mean reported?

2. For what group and what variable is the highest mean reported?

   a.   Group

   b.   Variable

3. Which measure of the marital variables is the most homogeneous (i.e., has the least variation)?

4. Which group (i.e., husbands or wives) was the most heterogeneous in reporting CFIDS symptoms?

5. The following is the text in which the researchers discuss the data in Table 4. Does the information in the table and the text agree? (*Note:* Ignore the $p < .01, p < .001$, and $p < .001$ notation.)

> "No significant differences were found in the couples' reported marital relationship variables of marital adjustment, marital empathy, marital support, and marital conflict. The paired wives' and husbands' descriptions of the wives' CFIDS symptoms, using the DCFSS, were significantly different. Wives' and husbands' reported number of symptoms . . . the mean problem scores . . . and the total problem scores . . . were significantly different." (Goodwin, 1997)

Check your answers with those in Appendix A, Chapter 14.

Activity 5

Using the studies in Appendices A-D in the textbook, answer the following questions regarding the use of descriptive statistics in each study. Once again, use the Critical Thinking Decision Path in Chapter 14 of the textbook.

1. Was the use of descriptive statistics appropriate for this study?

   a. Wikblad and Anderson

   b. Draucker and Petrovic

   c. Rudy et al

   d. Ward, Berry, and Misiewicz

2. Were descriptive statistics used in the study?

    a.   Wikblad and Anderson

    b.   Draucker and Petrovic

    c.   Rudy et al

    d.   Ward, Berry, and Misiewicz

3. What data were summarized and/or explained through the use of descriptive statistics?

    a.   Wikblad and Anderson

    b.   Draucker and Petrovic

    c.   Rudy et al

    d.   Ward, Berry, and Misiewicz

4. Were the descriptive statistics used appropriately?

    a.   Wikblad and Anderson

    b.   Draucker and Petrovic

    c.   Rudy et al

    d.   Ward, Berry, and Misiewicz

5. Which of the four studies relied the most heavily on the use of descriptive statistics?

Check your answers in Appendix A, Chapter 14.

Posttest

1. Two outpatient clinics measured client waiting time as one indicator of effectiveness. The mean and standard deviation of waiting time in minutes is reported below. Which outpatient clinic would you prefer, assuming that all other things are equal? Explain your answer.

	Clinic 1	Clinic 2
Mean (in minutes)	40	25
Standard deviation (in minutes)	10	45

2. You are responsible for ordering a new supply of hospital gowns for your unit. Which measure of central tendency would be the most useful in your decision making? Explain your answer.

3. Using Table 5 on the next page as the basis for your answers, answer the following questions.

    a.   How many total subjects participated in this study?

    b.   What advice would men most frequently give to someone newly diagnosed with human papillomavirus infection (HPV)?

    c.   Do the men and women agree about the advice they would be the most likely to give to someone newly diagnosed with HPV? Explain your answer.

Answers to the posttest items are in the *Instructor's Resource Manual*.
Check with your instructor for these answers.

Table 5. Types of Helpful Advice and Information

	n(%) Respondents	n(%) Women	n(%) Men
Balanced Perspective			
Maintain a positive outlook	39 (44)	27 (44)	12 (44)
Remember you are not alone	20 (23)	15 (25)	5 (19)
Avoid self-blame and negative self-evaluation	18 (21)	17 (28)	1 (4)
Remember that time will heal	8 (9)	8 (13)	0 (0)
Treatment			
Seek treatment for yourself	44 (50)	30 (49)	14 (52)
Realize that warts are treatable	9 (10)	6 (10)	3 (11)
Establish a positive relationship with health care provider	8 (9)	7 (11)	1 (4)
Be realistic about future course of disease	5 (6)	3 (5)	2 (7)
Check yourself for recurrences	3 (3)	2 (3)	1 (4)
Seek evaluation for partners	2 (2)	2 (3)	0 (0)
Sexual Behavior			
Practice safer sex	34 (39)	20 (33)	14 (52)
Inform sexual partners	14 (16)	11 (18)	3 (11)
Knowledge			
Educate yourself and ask questions	21 (24)	15 (25)	6 (22)
Expect inconsistent information	4 (5)	3 (5)	1 (4)
Self Care			
Seek emotional support	11 (13)	11 (18)	0 (0)
Maintain a healthy lifestyle	11 (13)	7 (11)	4 (15)
Other			
Not codable	8 (9)	6 (10)	2 (7)
Having genital warts did not affect me in any way	3 (3)	3 (5)	0 (0)
I don't know what to tell others	1 (1)	0 (0)	1 (4)

Taylor CA, Keller ML, Egan JJ: Advice from affected persons about living with human papillomavirus infection, Image: J Nurs Schol 29(1):27-32, 1997.

References

Baldwin KA, Chen SC: Use of public health nursing services: relationship to adequacy of prenatal care and infant outcome, *Public Health Nurs* 13(1):13-20, 1996.

Draucker B, Petrovic K: Healing of adult male survivors of childhood sexual abuse, *Image: J Nurs Schol* 28:325-330, 1996.

Goodwin SS: The marital relationship and health in women with chronic fatigue and immune dysfunction syndrome: views of wives and husbands, *Nurs Res* 46(3):138-146, 1997.

Johnson JE: Social support and physical health in the rural elderly, *Appl Nurs Res* 9(2):61-66, 1996.

Lipp EJ, Deane D, Trimbe N: Cardiovascular disease risks in adolescent males, *Appl Nurs Res* 9(3):102-107, 1996.

McFarlane J, Parker B, Soeken K: Abuse during pregnancy: associations with maternal health and infant birth weight, *Nurs Res* 45(1):37-42, 1996.

Rudy EB et al: Patient outcomes for the chronically critically ill: special care unit versus intensive care unit, *Nurs Res* 44:324-331, 1995.

Taylor CA, Keller ML, Egan JJ: Advice from affected persons about living with human papillomavirus infection, *Image: J Nurs Schol* 29(1):27-32, 1997.

Ward SE, Berry PE, Misiewicz H: Concerns about analgesics among patients and family caregivers in a hospice setting, *Res Nurs Health* 19:205-211, 1996.

Wikblad K, Anderson B: A comparison of three wound dressings in patients undergoing heart surgery, *Nurs Res* 44:312-316, 1995.

Wineman NM et al: Relationships among illness uncertainty, stress, coping, and emotional well-being at entry into a clinical drug trial, *Appl Nurs Res* 9(2):53-60, 1996.

Inferential Data Analysis

15

Kathleen Rose-Grippa

Introduction

Descriptive statistics are valuable for summarizing data and allowing us to look at salient features about a group of data, but practitioners usually want more information. They want to be able to read about an intervention used with a specific group of individuals and consider the usefulness of that intervention with the clients in their care. These decisions require practitioners to be comfortable with the assumption that the clients in the study and the clients in their care are members of the same population and that the clinical outcomes are a result of the intervention. The researcher's use of inferential statistics in the data analysis is one strategy for building confidence in that critical assumption.

Initially, the numbers, symbols, and tables used to present inferential statistics are intimidating. You can take several steps to reduce that intimidation factor: Take a deep breath and jump in. Remember you have the intelligence and the skills to do this. Learn to look at the array of numbers and symbols one step at a time. Continue to read clinically relevant research. This chapter is designed to help you with the skills part of the task. We will spend a bit of time reviewing the logic underlying inferential statistics, take a look at some specific inferential tools, and spend the bulk of our effort digesting data from the studies included in the text.

Learning Outcomes

On completion of this chapter, the student should be able to do the following:
* Identify the symbols representing specified inferential statistical techniques.
* Choose an appropriate inferential statistical strategy for specified research hypotheses.
* Interpret the results of specified inferential statistical tests.
* Critique the use of inferential statistics in given studies.

Activity 1

Shortcuts are wonderful. Memorizing the statistical notation saves a lot of time that would be spent flipping through pages looking for the symbol.

The following lists the inferential statistical tools as they appear in Figure 15-1 in the textbook (before beginning this activity, read through the list):

Technique	Notation
Pearson product moment correlation	r
Phi coefficient	ϕ
Kendall's tau	τ
Spearman rho	rs
Multiple regression	R
Path analysis	None used
Canonical correlation	Rc
Contingency coefficient	None used
Discriminant function analysis	None used
Logistic regression	None used
t-test	t
ANOVA	F
Chi-square	χ^2
Signed rank	Z
Mann Whitney U	U

Now, obtain the following supplies: a package of 3 x 5 index cards, preferably lined on one side; six pens or a combination of pens and highlighters that will give you six different colors; one broad-tipped, black-ink marker.

You are to create your own set of "statistical assistants." Once they are finished carry them with you when you go to the library. Use them when you are reading reports of research. Before long you will be able to read a piece of research without referring to your stack of statistical assistants.

Once this activity is completed, you will have a set of quick reference cards and a set of flash cards that can be used for memorization exercises.

1. Make your key card first. Take one of the cards and on the side without lines, using the broad-tipped, black marker write *NAME OF INFERENTIAL STATISTICAL TECHNIQUE.*

2. Turn the card over and use the side with lines. Choose one of the pens with colored ink and, on the first line, write *Symbol.* Complete this side of the card with five more categories of information using a different line and a different color of ink for each line for each category. The lined side of the card should look like this:

Symbol

# of independent variables (IV)   # of dependent variables (DV)

IV's level of measurement

DV's level of measurement

HR = relationship? (# of variables?)   differences? (# of groups?)

Parametric/nonparametric

Of course, your card will look prettier because each line of your key card will be in a different color. Now let's move on to creating your stack of statistical assistants.

3. On the front of each card (side without lines) write the full name of one of the inferential statistical tools. Use the broad-tipped, black marker to do this. For example, *Pearson product moment correlation.*

4. Turn the card over and write the information that corresponds to the appropriate category on the key card in the appropriate line using the appropriate color of ink. For example, the lined side of the Pearson product moment correlation card would read as follows:

r

IV = 1 DV = 1

IV = at least interval

DV = at least interval

Relationship (2 variables)

Parametric

Check your answers with those in Appendix A, Chapter 15.

Activity 2

Let's practice using some of the inferential techniques listed in Activity 1. Below is a list of some studies that have used some of the statistical techniques listed in Activity 1. The specific technique is listed at the end of the citation in bold type.

Duffy M, Rossow R, Hernandez M: Correlates of health-promotion activities in employed Mexican American women, *Nurs Res* 45(1):18-24, 1996. **Canonical correlation**

Hall LA et al: Self-esteem as a mediator of the effects of stressors and social resources on depressive symptoms in postpartum mothers, *Nurs Res* 45(4):231-238, 1996. **Multiple regression, multiple logistic regression, path analysis**

Jacobsen BS, Munro BH, Brooten DA: Comparison of original and revised scoring systems for the Multiple Affect Adjective Check List, *Nurs Res* 45(1):57-60, 1996. **Mann-Whitney and Kruskal-Wallis**

Miller AM, Champion VL: Mammography in older women: one-time and three-year adherence to guidelines, *Nurs Res* 45(4):239-245, 1996. **Logistic regression**

Purath J, Lansinger T, Ragheb C: Cardiac risk evaluation for elementary school children, *Public Health Nurs* 12(3):189-195, 1995. **Pearson correlation coefficient**

Ronen T, Abraham Y: Retention control training in the treatment of younger versus older enuretic children, *Nurs Res* 45(2):78-82, 1996. **t-test and ANOVA**

Tripp-Reimer T et al: The dimensional structure of nursing interventions, *Nurs Res* 45(1):10-17, 1996. **Canonical correlation**

Activity 3

We'll walk through the thinking used in inferential statistics with examples from the studies that are included in the text. The researcher's choice of which inferential statistic to use is the result of a fairly long chain of decisions. The decisions begin with the researcher's formulation of the questions that are operating in the clinical setting: If I do this, will it make a difference? If I take this action, will I see a change in the client's status? The decisions regarding research design, sampling strategies, and available data collection instruments follow. All of these decisions lead the researcher to the choice of analytical strategies which would include the choice of inferential statistical techniques.

Let's walk through the Wikblad and Anderson (1995) study while thinking about these decisions.

1. What was the basic question addressed by Wikblad and Anderson?
   Take a close look at the second sentence of the second paragraph and the paragraph immediately preceding the section labeled *Methods*.

2. Is the research hypothesis written or implied?

3. Write, using your own words, the research hypothesis.

4. Write the null hypothesis.

5. What function does the null hypothesis serve?

6. Identify the variables that are identified by the researchers.

   Independent Variable(s)   **Dependent Variable(s)**

7. Does the question/research hypothesis/null hypothesis address "differences among groups" or "a relationship between variables"?

8. How many categories of the independent variable exist?

9. What level of measurement was used to measure the dependent variable(s)?

10. Use your "statistical assistant" cards. Which inferential technique do you think was appropriate?

11. Check the study. Is this the one Wikblad and Anderson used?

12. Find the Results section of the study. Within this section find the paragraphs which discuss the patients' discomfort when the dressings were removed (subsection is entitled *Removal of the Dressing*). Read the second paragraph that begins "Pain at removal . . ." Imagine yourself as a patient in this study. Based on the information in this paragraph what kind of dressing would you want on your incision? Explain your answer.

13. Think through and write out the clinical significance of having committed a Type I error in terms of the "pain at removal" data.

Check your answers with those in Appendix A, Chapter 15.

Activity 4

This activity consists of a series of interpretations. The best way to become comfortable with inferential statistics is to work with them. The process can be slow and tedious, but remember how awkward you felt the first time you helped a patient with a variety of attachments move from one location to another. You practiced. Transferring became easier, so will the reading and interpretation of statistics.

1. Refer to the Rudy et al (1995) study in the textbook, and find the Method section. The sample is the first subheading in this section. The third paragraph begins: "To ensure similarity in acuity of illness . . ." and goes on to explain that the "experimental and control groups were equivalent." Why would this be important information in this study?

2. Look at Table 2 in the Rudy et al study. For what outcome was there statistically significant results?

3. Explain why the chi-square statistic was used to analyze the data regarding "discharge disposition from hospital." (Refer to Table 2 of the Rudy et al study in the textbook.)

4. The next two items are to be answered using Table 1 from the Bucher et al study reprinted below (*Note:* LBW = low birth weight; NBW = normal birth weight).

   a.   What two barriers were statistically significant?

   b.   What are your thoughts regarding the clinical implications of this one finding?

Table 1. Differences in Barriers to Prenatal Care Services by Infant Birth Weight Group

Barriers to Prenatal Care Services	Mothers of LBW Infants (n = 43)	Mothers of NBW Infants (n = 98)	
	M	M	t
Transportation	1.5	1.0	2.49*
Cost of traveling	1.4	1.1	1.84
Other financial problems	1.6	1.2	2.50*
Length of travel time	1.3	1.2	0.53
Clinic/doctor's office hours	1.4	1.3	0.54
Child care	1.0	1.1	0.74
Language/cultural differences	1.1	1.0	1.53
Alcohol or substance abuse	1.1	1.0	1.12
Understanding of information	1.1	1.1	1.13
Timing of pregnancy	1.2	1.1	1.01

Higher ratings indicate the barrier was more of a problem
*$p < .02$

From Butcher et al: First time mother's perceptions of prenatal care services, Appl Nurs Res 10(2):64-71, 1997.

5. Use Table 2, which is reprinted on the next page from the Failla et al study, to address the next set of items.

   a. One reads in the narrative of the study: "A significant negative correlation was indicated between hopelessness and health-related hardiness, while a significant positive correlation was indicated between hopelessness and uncertainty." What are the specific correlations in each pair of variables?

   b. Using your own words, what do these statistically significant correlations mean?

   c. Which correlations in Table 2 do you find the most interesting? What intrigues you?

6. Table 3, which is reprinted below from the Failla et al study, provides information regarding the use of a stepwise multiple regression analysis with these data. Use the discussion in the text regarding multiple regression and take a stab at interpreting this table.

Table 3. Stepwise Multiple Regression Analysis of Predictor Variables of Adjustment

Predictor Variables	Beta	R^2	R^2 Change	F	p
Hopelessness	2.85	.387	.387	17.03	.0003
Income	3.03	.527	.140	7.68	.0102

From Failla S et al: Adjustment of women with systemic lupus erythematosus, Appl Nurs Res 9(2):87-93, 1996.

Table 2. Pearson Correlations Between Study Variables

Variable	Education	Income	MUIS-C	BHI	HRHS	HRHS-C	HRHS-C/C
Income	.39*						
MUIS-C	-.41*	-.16					
BHI -	.26	.10	.46**				
HRHS	.05	-.05	-.17	-.63***			
Control	.002	-.24	-.33	-.60**	.77****		
Commitment/challenge	.07	.08	-.03	-.51**	.90****	.42*	
PAIS	.32	.33	-.53**	-.62***	.30	.24	.20
Health care orientation	.10	-.05	-.42*	-.32	.16	.34	.003
Vocation	.09	.24	-.33	-.49**	.28	.12	.32
Domestic	.35*	.48**	-.47**	-.43*	.13	.19	.06
Social relations	.23	.32	.03	-.08	.05	-.09	.13
Sexual relations	.29	.18	-.34	-.44*	.33	.24	.30
Extended family relationships	.35*	.26	-.39*	-.63**	.39*	.27	.36*
Psychological distress	.20	.17	-.39*	-.64****	.22	.17	.20

MUIS-C, Mishel Uncertainty in Illness-Community Form; BHI, Beck Hopelessness Index; HRHS, Health-Related Hardiness Scale; PAIS, Psychological Adjustment to Illness Scale.
*p ≤ .05; **p ≤ .01; ***p ≤ .001; ****p ≤ .0001.

From Failla S et al: Adjustment of women with systemic lupus erythematosus, Appl Nurs Res 9(2):87-93, 1996.

7. Table 4 from the LoBiondo-Wood et al study is reproduced on the next page. Look at the numbers in the table. Which pairs of numbers would you initially wonder if they were statistically significant?

Check your answers with those in Appendix A, Chapter 15.

Posttest

1. The use of a Pearson correlation coefficient and analysis of variance indicates that the variable was measured on which of the following?
    a.   Nominal scale
    b.   Ordinal scale
    c.   Interval or ratio scale

2. Indicate whether the following values are statistically significant or not statistically significant. Use A to indicate statistically significant and B to indicate not statistically significant. Remember that critical table values are those at the relevant point on the normal distribution curve.

   a.   _____ $t = 2.03$, df = 38, p = .01, critical table value is 2.42

   b.   _____ $F(2,20) = 2.67$, p = .05, critical table value is 3.49

   c.   _____ $\chi^2 = 13.07$, df = 2, p = .05, critical table value is 5.99

   d.   _____ $F(3,16) = 19.20$, p = .01, critical table value is 5.29

   e.   _____ $t = 6.79$, df = 58, p = .05, critical table value is 1.67

Table 4. QLI & Subscales for Means & Standard Deviation

	Time I PRETX		Time II 3 Months		Time III 6 Months		Time IV 12 Months		Time V 18 Months	
	M	SD	M	SD	M	SD	M	SD	M	SD
QLI total	19.3	4.7	23.3	3.7	23.7	4.6	24.0	4.3	22.9	4.4
HF	15.2	7.3	23.5	4.4	24.3	5.0	24.4	4.7	22.7	5.5
SE	21.6	4.1	21.6	3.4	22.0	4.6	23.0	4.5	21.9	4.3
PS	18.6	6.6	23.8	5.3	23.8	5.3	23.5	5.2	23.0	4.9
F	26.2	3.7	26.0	4.2	25.8	4.8	25.8	4.5	25.6	4.9

Abbreviations. QLI, quality of life; HF, health and functioning; SE, socioeconomic; PS, Psychological/spiritual; F, family.

From LoBiondo-Wood G et al: Impact of liver transplant on quality of life: a longitudinal perspective, Appl Nurs Res 10(1):27-32, 1997.

3. Use Table 5 from the Chappell, Dickey, and DeLetter study reprinted below to answer the last items.

   a. Which type of medication error occurred most frequently?

   b. Can you find the arithmetic error in the table?

   c. The experimental group in this study used medication dispensers. Would you advise that this practice be adopted in other residential caregiver situations? Why or why not?

Table 5. Mean Medication Errors per Patient in Residential Care Homes

	Control group mean (n = 46)	Experimental group mean (n = 32)	t-	p
Duplications	.78	.28	1.21	ns
Omissions	2.46	.66	1.87	.06*
Total	3.23	.94	2.22	.03*

From Chappell HW, Dickey C, DeLotta M: The use of medication dispensers in residential care homes, Family Comm Health 20(2):48:57, 1997.

The answers to the posttest are in the *Instructor's Resource Manual*.
Please check with your instructor for these answers.

References

Bucher L et al: First-time mothers' perceptions of prenatal care services, *Appl Nurs Res* 10(2):64-71, 1997.

Chappell HW, Dickey C, DeLetter M: The use of medication dispensers in residential care homes, *Family Comm Health* 20(2):48-57, 1997.

Duffy M, Rossow R, Hernandez M: Correlates of health-promotion activities in employed Mexican American women, *Nurs Res* 45(1):18-24, 1996.

Failla S et al: Adjustment of women with systemic lupus erythematosus, *Appl Nurs Res* 9(2):87-93, 1996.

Hall LA et al: Self-esteem as a mediator of the effects of stressors and social resources on depressive symptoms in postpartum mothers, *Nurs Res* 45(4):231-238, 1996.

Jacobsen BS, Munro BH, Brooten DA: Comparison of original and revised scoring systems for the Multiple Affect Adjective Check List, *Nurs Res* 45(1):57-60, 1996.

LoBiondo-Wood G et al: Impact of liver transplantation on quality of life: a longitudinal perspective, *Appl Nurs Res* 10(1):27-32, 1997.

Miller AM, Champion VL: Mammography in older women: One-time and three-year adherence to guidelines, *Nurs Res* 45(4):239-245, 1996.

Purath J, Lansinger T, Ragheb C: Cardiac risk evaluation for elementary school children, *Public Health Nurs* 12(3):189-195, 1995.

Ronen T, Abraham Y: Retention control training in the treatment of younger versus older enuretic children, *Nurs Res* 45(2):78-82, 1996.

Rudy EB et al: Patient outcomes for the chronically critically ill: special care unit versus intensive care unit, *Nurs Res* 44(6):324-331, 1995.

Tripp-Reimer T et al: The dimensional structure of nursing interventions, *Nurs Res* 45(1):10-17, 1996.

Wikblad K, Anderson B: A comparison of three wound dressings in patients undergoing heart surgery, *Nurs Res* 44(5):312-316, 1995.

Analysis of the Findings *16*

Sharon S. Mullen

Introduction

As the last sections of a research report, the results and conclusions sections answer the question "So what?" In other words, it is in these two sections that the investigator "makes sense" of the research, critically synthesizes the data, ties them to a theoretical framework, and builds on a body of knowledge. These two sections are a very important part of the research report because they describe the generalizability of the findings and offer recommendations for further research. Well-written, clear, and concise results and conclusions sections provide valuable information for nursing practice. Conversely, poorly written results and conclusions sections will leave a reader bewildered, confused, and wondering how or if the findings are relevant to nursing.

Learning Outcomes

On completion of this chapter, the student should be able to do the following:
- Know the difference between the results sections of a study and the discussion sections of the study.
- Interpret table and figure findings from a research report.
- Describe various generalizations and limitations of a research report
- Synthesize data and identify implications for nursing.
- Identify recommendations from a research report.

Activity 1

Knowing what information to look for and where to find it in the Results and Discussions sections of a research report will enable you to interpret the research findings and critique research reports.

1. Identify the section in which the following information from the research report may be found. Put an *A* in the blank space if the information would be found in the Results section and a *B* if the information would be found in the Discussion section.

   a. _____ Tables/figures

   b. _____ Limitations of the study

   c. _____ Data analysis related to the literature review

   d. _____ Inferences or generalization of results

   e. _____ Statistical support or non-support of hypotheses

   f. _____ Findings of the hypothesis testing

   g. _____ Information about the statistical tests used to analyze hypotheses

   h. _____ Application of meaning (makes sense) of data analysis

   i. _____ Suggestions for further research

   j. _____ Recommendations for nursing practice

2. Read the results and discussion sections of the study *A Comparison of Three Wound Dressings in Patients Undergoing Heart Surgery* by Wikblad and Anderson (1995) found in Appendix A of the text. Respond to the following questions.

   a. Wound healing effectiveness did not differ among the three types of wound dressings.
   True   False

   b. When patients in the hydroactive dressing group were compared with patients in the absorbent dressing group, a chi-square statistical analysis revealed patients receiving the absorbent dressing had statistically significant better healing rates.
   True   False

c. No statistically significant difference in wound healing effectiveness was found between the hydrocolloid and the absorbent dressing groups.
True   False

d. Comparing ease with which dressings are removed, nurses reported no statistically significant difference among the three types of dressings.
True   False

e. According to the study findings, the hydroactive dressing was significantly more painful to the patient when removed.
True   False

3. Discuss the implications for nursing from the results of the Wikblad and Anderson study. Assuming you are a nurse manager on a coronary care unit, and have the option of using one of the three types of dressing examined in the study, explain which dressing you might use and why.

4. Interpret the following statistical findings from Wikblad and Anderson's study.

a. Comparing redness in wounds on the fifth postoperative day between the hydroactive dressing group and the absorbent dressing group, a chi-square statistical test revealed a statistic of X^2 (2, n = 153) = 17.8, p < 0.0001. What conclusion may be reached from this finding?

b. Interpret the following chi-square test result in comparing wound redness between the hydrocolloid dressing group and the absorbent dressing group X^2 (2, n = 150) = 4.1, p > 05.

c. Identify the components of the following statistical test result taken from Wikblad and Anderson's article. X^2 (6, n = 213) = 33.0, p < 0.0001.

1. X^2 _____   a. Sample size

2. 6   _____   b. Degrees of freedom

3. n = 213 _____   c. Chi-square symbol

4. 33.0   _____   d. Probability level

5. p < 0.0001 _____   e. Chi-square test statistic

d. When a probability level is calculated as p < 0.05 and the researcher has previously set the alpha level of significance at 0.05, the researcher must reject the null hypothesis and accept the alternate hypothesis.
True   False

e. If a researcher calculates a probability level of p > 0.05 and rejects the null hypothesis in favor of the alternate hypothesis, the researcher has made a Type I error.
True   False

Check your answers with those in Appendix A, Chapter 16.

Activity 2

Interpreting qualitative research results and conclusions differ significantly from quantitative research findings. After reading the article by Draucker and Petrovic (1996), *Healing of Adult Male Survivors of Childhood Sexual Abuse* found in Appendix B of the text, complete the following items.

1. The researchers identified a theoretical framework based on the analysis of the data obtained from the subjects. The researchers report that subjects described their childhood sexual abuse survival as a journey. Briefly explain the authors' theoretical framework.

2. Read the summary and conclusion sections of Draucker and Petrovic's article and list three to five implications for nursing in caring for adult male clients who have been sexually abused.

   a.

   b.

   c.

   d.

   e.

3. Draucker and Petrovic studied male survivors of childhood sexual abuse. Identify two to three suggestions for further research based on these findings.

   a.

   b.

   c.

Check your answers with those in Appendix A, Chapter 16.

Activity 3

Being able to interpret tables in research articles is an important part of the critiquing process. Read Ward, Berry, and Misiewicz's (1996) article *Concerns About Analgesics Among Patients and Family Caregivers in a Hospice Setting*, found in Appendix D of the textbook, and answer the following items.

1. The following items pertain to Table 1 of the article.

   a. Which two groups comprise the subjects for the study?

   b. What is the total number of married subjects for both groups?
      1. 21   2. 28   3. 35   4. 49

c. Which group has a higher percentage of subjects who have had more than a high-school education?

    1. Patient   2. Caregiver

d. In a narrative sentence describe the demographic characteristics of the subjects by interpreting Table 1.

2. Use Table 2 of the Ward, Berry, and Misiewicz article to answer the following items.

   a. What is the alpha level of significance set by the researchers for the study?

     1. 0.05   2. 0.01   3. 0.001   4. 0.0001

   b. Table 2 reports correlation scores between a pair of variables on several subscales. For example, the patient and caregiver were asked in the BQ to identify their fear of addiction. The correlation coefficient for this variable was 0.36. It was not significant, meaning there was no statistically significant relationship between the patients' and caregivers' fear of addiction. There was a statistically significant relationship between the patients' and caregivers' scores on one subscale. Using Table 2, which one is it?

     1. Fear of injections
     2. Desires to be a good patient
     3. Concern about drug tolerance
     4. Fatalism about pain relief

   c. There is a statistically significant relationship (correlation) between BQ total score between patient and caregiver as identified in Table 2.

     True   False

   d. What are the implications for nursing based on the results of the findings in Table 2? (*Hint:* Look back to research question (a) in the study.)

3. Research question (b) in the study asks who has greater concerns about reporting pain and using analgesics, the patient or the caregiver? Table 3 addresses this question. Review Table 3 and answer the following items.

   a. There is a statistically significant difference between patient and caregiver on the BQ total score (t = 0.92).

     True   False

b. Which variable indicates a statistically significant difference between patient and care-giver?
    1. Fear of injections
    2. Desire to be a good patient
    3. Fatalism about pain relief
    4. Concern about side effects

c. Based on the research findings, what conclusions may be reached regarding research question (b) in the study?

4. The discussion section of the Ward, Berry, and Misiewicz article is quite lengthy. After reading it, identify three to five implications for nursing based on the findings and conclusions of the study.

a.

b.

c.

d.

e.

Check your answers with those in Appendix A, Chapter 16.

Activity 4

The overall differences between the intensive care unit (ICU) and the special care unit (SCU) is the focus of the Rudy et al (1995) article *Patient Outcomes for the Chronically Critically Ill: Special Care Unit Versus Intensive Care Unit* found in Appendix C of the text. Read the article, focusing particularly on the Results and Discussion sections, and complete the following items.

1. Identify the authors' purpose of the study.

2. The two groups in the study SCU versus ICU were compared on six different variables. List these variables.

   a.

   b.

   c.

   d.

   e.

   f.

3. The researchers used two statistical tests to analyze the data. Name them.

4. Tables 2 and 3 answer the initial purpose of the study. One variable, however, is not identified on either one of the tables. Which one is it?
   1. Mortality
   2. Length of stay
   3. Cost
   4. Patient and family satisfaction

5. One finding dealt with patient and family satisfaction. Results indicated no differences in levels of patient and family satisfaction between the ICU or the SCU groups. More specifically, what was the level of satisfaction for both groups (ICU and SCU)?
   a. Patients and family were somewhat dissatisfied.
   b. Patients and family were highly dissatisfied.
   c. Patients and family were somewhat satisfied.
   d. Patients and family were highly satisfied.

6. As a nurse manager of the ICU, you have read the study by Rudy et al. You note you have no available beds on your unit and some patients will have to be transferred to the SCU to make room for critically ill patients. The nursing staff fears that the SCU is unable to deliver quality care to critically ill patients in the same manner as the ICU. Based on the findings of Rudy et al, what rationale could you provide to your staff to ease their concerns?

Check your answers with those in Appendix A, Chapter 16.

Posttest

1. When a research hypothesis is supported through testing, it may be assumed that the hypothesis was which of the following?
   a. Proved
   b. Accepted
   c. Rejected
   d. Disconfirmed

2. Limitations of a study describe its weaknesses.
   True   False

3. The Results section of a research study includes all the following except:
   a. Hypothesis testing results
   b. Tables and figures
   c. Statistical test description
   d. Limitations of the study

4. Unsupported hypotheses mean that the study is of little value in generating knowledge.
   True   False

5. Tables in research reports should meet all of the following criteria except:
   a. Clear, concise tables
   b. Restate the text narrative
   c. Economize the text
   d. Supplement the text narrative

6. The discussion section provides opportunity for the investigator to do all of the following except:
   a. Describe implications from the research results
   b. Relate the results to the literature review
   c. Make generalizations to large populations of subjects
   d. Suggest areas for further research

7. Hypothesis testing is described in the discussion section of the research report.
   True   False

The answers to the posttest are in the *Instructor's Resource Manual.*
Please check with your instructor for these answers.

References

Draucker C, Petrovic K: Healing of adult male survivors of childhood sexual abuse, *Image: J Nurs Schol* 28(4):325-330, 1996.

Rudy E et al: Patient outcomes for the chronically critically ill: special care unit versus intensive care unit, *Nurs Res* 44(6):324-331, 1995.

Ward S, Berry P, Misiewicz H: Concerns about analgesics among patients and family caregiver in a hospice setting, *Res Nurs Health* 19:205-211, 1996.

Wikblad K, Anderson B; A comparison of three wound dressings in patients undergoing heart surgery, *Nurs Res* 44(5):312-316, 1995.

Evaluating Quantitative Research Studies

17

Kathleen Rose-Grippa

Introduction

Now is the time for you to put together all of the pieces that you have studied throughout this book. Read through the studies and the written critiques that are part of Chapter 17 in the textbook.

A useful way of doing this is as follows:

1. Read the research report from beginning to end. Do not stop to puzzle over this particular piece or that particular section. Just start at the beginning and read to the end. This will give you an impression of the article as a whole.

2. Read through the critiquing guidelines found in Table 17-1 of the textbook.

3. Read the journal article again. This time jot down any thoughts that might occur to you while reading. The margins of the book or those of the copy of the journal article are easy places to note thoughts that you want to review again.

4. Now go through the article section by section. Read the questions from Table 17-1, then read the relevant section of the research report. Answer the questions. The answers to these questions will become the working draft of the written critique.

5. Now write in narrative style the critique you have just finished thinking through. Be careful with your use of language. Do not be brutal, but do raise any questions that you have.

Learning Outcomes

On completion of this chapter, the student should be able to do the following:
* Practice thinking through a critique.
* Practice writing a critique.

Activity 1

The exercise for this chapter is to practice thinking through a critique. The two critiques presented in the text will give you a sense of style, length, and flow. After you have read them, read the Wikblad and Anderson study with the intent of writing a critique. Use the steps listed above. Write a first draft of a critique.

Problem Statement and Purpose

Review of Literature and Theoretical Framework

Hypotheses or Research Questions

Sample

Research Design

Internal Validity

External Validity

Methods

Legal-Ethical Issues

Instruments

Reliability and Validity

Analysis of Data

Conclusions, Implications, and Recommendations

(The answers in Appendix A, Chapter 17 will not provide you with a written critique, but they will give you the answers to the questions listed in the critiquing guidelines table in Chapter 17.)

Note: There is no posttest available for this chapter . . . Enjoy the break!

Evaluating the Qualitative Research Report 18

Sharon A. Denham

Introduction

Qualitative research provides an opportunity to generate new knowledge about phenomena less easily studied with empirical or quantitative methods. Nurse researchers increasingly are using qualitative methods to explore holistic aspects less easily understood with only objective measures. The important contributions being made to nursing knowledge through qualitative studies make it important for nurses to possess skills for critiquing and evaluating qualitative research reports.

Learning Outcomes

On completion of this chapter, the student should be able to do the following:
- Identify the influence of stylistic considerations on the presentation of a qualitative research report.
- Identify the criteria for critiquing a qualitative research report.
- Evaluate the strengths and weaknesses of a qualitative research report.
- Describe the applicability of the findings of a qualitative research report.

Activity 1

The methods of presentation in qualitative research reports are different than those in quantitative studies. Nurses doing qualitative research reports are challenged to present the richness of the data within the restrictions of publication guidelines.

Review the article entitled *Healing of Adult Male Survivors of Childhood Sexual Abuse* (Draucker and Petrovic, 1996) to identify the ways the researchers stylistically presented the rich data (see Appendix B in the textbook).

1. In the finding section entitled *Living in the Dungeon*, the researchers described three aspects of this experience and gave examples from the data to describe what is meant by the descriptive terms used. Read through this section and find an example of the data that defines each term.

    a. *Being confined*:

    b. *Being trapped*:

    c. *Being silenced*:

    d. *Being stifled*:

    e. *Being idled*:

Check your answers with those in Appendix A, Chapter 18.

Activity 2

The findings of qualitative studies describe or explain a phenomenon within a specific context. The findings are usually not generalizable to other groups, which means that persons who want to apply the findings to others have the responsibility to validate whether the findings are applicable in a different setting with other groups.

The theory described by Drauker and Petrovic (1996) is that the healing of adult male survivors of sexual abuse involves an internal force (struggling against emotional pain) and an external force (the societal view that men should not be victims).

1. Identify two factors you would want to consider if you intended to apply these findings to other groups of adult men who had been victims of sexual abuse.

2. Explain what it means to be "context bound."

3. Identify how the subject population in the Drauker and Petrovic (1996) study might be considered context bound and what implications this might have if the study was to be replicated.

4. Qualitative research is also used to examine important concepts. What is the concept this study adds to the existing body of knowledge?

5. Instrument development is another way findings from qualitative studies are used. How might the findings from the Drauker and Petrovic (1996) study be applied to sexual abuse of males?

Check your answers with those in Appendix A, Chapter 18.

Activity 3

Critiquing qualitative research enables the nurse to make sense out of the research report, build on the body of knowledge about human phenomena, and consider how knowledge might be applicable to nursing. Learning and applying a critiquing process is the first step in this process.

1. Review Table 18-1 in the textbook and answer the following. Match the qualitative research process in Column A with the activity in Column B. Some steps are used more than once.

Column A

A. Subject selection

B. Study method

C. Researcher perspective

D. Data analysis

E. Application of findings

F. Findings description

G. Study design

Column B

a. _____ The purpose of the study is clearly stated.

b. _____ Audio-taped interviews were used to collect phenomenological data.

c. _____ Do the participants recognize the experience as their own?

d. _____ Purposive sampling was used.

e. _____ Data are clearly reported in the research report

f. _____ The researcher has remained true to the findings.

g. _____ Recommendations for future research are made.

h. _____ The phenomenon of interest is clearly identified.

i. _____ Participant observation was done in an ethnography.

2. In Chapter 9 of the textbook, locate Table 9-5, which is entitled *Criteria for Judging Scientific Rigor*. Use this table to answer the following items about the Drauker and Petrovic (1996) study about male sexual abuse.

    a.   Describe what you view as the credibility of the study findings:

    b.   Explain what you perceive as the auditability of the findings:

    c.   Discuss your perceptions about the fittingness of the findings:

Check your answers with those in Appendix A, Chapter 18.

Activity 4

The Scannell-Desch article entitled *The Lived Experience of Women Military Nurses in Vietnam During the Vietnam War*, in Chapter 18 of the textbook used phenomenology to study the lived experience of nurses during a war. The participants served during the war from 1965 to 1973 and the majority were volunteers. The data collection for this study was conducted at least 20 years after having the war experience. As you think about the design of this study, think about how you would evaluate the findings and critique the study as you address the following.

Critique the study using the guidelines from the chapter in the textbook. Identify two concerns about the study that you might discuss with the investigator if provided an opportunity.

 Statement of the Phenomenon of Interest

Purpose

Method

Sampling

Data Collection

Data Analysis

Credibility

Auditability

Fittingness

Findings

Conclusions, Implications, and Recommendations

Check your answers with those in Appendix A, Chapter 18.

Posttest

1. True False   Qualitative research findings are generalizable to other groups.

2. True False   Findings from qualitative research designs are viewed as less credible by nurse researchers than those gained from quantitative studies.

3. True False   Auditability is an important aspect of evaluating a qualitative research report.

4. True False   The style of a qualitative research report differs from that of a quantitative research report.

5. True False   Some journal publication guidelines may impede the qualitative researcher's ability to convey the richness of the data.

6. True False   Journal reviewer's guidelines usually allow for the extra pages that qualitative researchers might need to provide the detail of their rich data.

7. _____ means that others should be able to identify the thinking, decisions, and methods used by the researcher when they conducted the research study.

8. _____ means that the study findings fit well outside the study situation.

9. _____ means that the research informants can identify the reported findings as their own experience.

10. _____ is the term usually applied to qualitative research to judge the validity and reliability of qualitative data.

References

Drauker CB, Petrovic K: Healing of adult male survivors of childhood sexual abuse, *Image: J Nurs Schol* 28(4):325-330, 1996.

Scannel-Desch EA: The lived experience of women military nurses in Vietnam during the Vietnam War, *Image: J Nurs Schol* 28(2):119-124, 1996.

Use of Research in Practice

19

Joy Edwards-Beckett

Introduction

Research is important to the clinician as a means to support current practice or to provide data to support a practice change. When using research to support or change practice, the clinician should consider two main aspects. First, what interventions provide the best patient outcomes? If there is no difference in patient outcomes when considering two or more interventions, then cost, in both dollars and time should also be considered. Second, if there is research support for a practice change, what process should the clinician follow for implementation?

Learning Outcomes

On completion of this chapter, the student should be able to do the following:
- Interpret a summary table to determine recommendations for practice.
- Identify organizational forces that affect research utilization.
- Evaluate an individual research study for its potential for utilization in the student's clinical setting.

Activity 1

Table 1 summarizes the findings from three studies on the use of heparin versus saline as a flush solution for peripheral intravenous locks of adult patients. Use the information in the table to respond to the items that follow.

1. With the information you have available, does each study meet the criteria for a sound study? Yes No

Table 1. Summary Table for Synthesis of Peripheral Lock Flush Solutions

Citation	Purpose/ Research Question	Sample Size	Variables & Measures		Statistical Tests	Significance Level	Results	Implications
			Independent	Dependent				
Geritz (1992)	To compare the efficacy of saline	150 peripheral IV lock sites versus 10 U/ml heparin flush solutions in peripheral IV locks	Saline versus heparin flush in 90 adults	Patency, reasons for solutions	Chi-square t-tests doing lock	p > 0.05	No difference in patency or reasons to discontinue lock	Recommend saline as flush—maintains same patient outcomes at lower cost
Peterson & Kirchnoff (1991)	To compare the efficacy of saline	20 research studies versus multiple heparin flush solutions in peripheral IV locks	Saline versus heparin flush (1 pediatric, 19 adult)	Patency phlebitis solutions	Meta-analysis of 13 studies that met criteria	d-index values z-scores significance not reached	No difference in phlebitis rates or loss of patency	Small number of pediatric studies, cannot extrapolate to children did not address cost issues
Shoaf & Oliver (1992)	To compare the efficacy of saline versus 10 U/ml heparin flush solutions in peripheral IV locks	260 adult surgical patients	Saline versus heparin flush solutions	Patency, phlebitis	Randomized blind 2-group design	95% Confidence intervals	No difference in patency or phlebitis	Recommend saline asflushing solution, did not calculate cost differences

2. How do the samples compare in the three studies? Are the patients comparable or different? Are the sample sizes sufficient?

3. How do the independent and dependent variables in the three studies compare? Are the researchers studying the same variables?

4. Compare and contrast the results of the three studies. Do they reach the same or different conclusions?

5. When examining the overall implications of the three studies, do they strongly support a particular flushing solution and flush method for peripheral locks? Why or why not? What flush solution do the studies recommend for practice?

Use Table 1 and the additional material from the studies included below in answering these questions.

Nursing Implications and Conclusions

Based on this study of 260 subjects, there were no significant differences in patency and phlebitis between the use of flushing solutions with normal saline versus a control of 10 U/mL heparin in normal saline injection to maintain an intermittent indwelling intravenous site. The study identified that the use of saline solution alone is less irritating and less expensive. Patients no longer incur the $4 charge for a heparin saline flush. These results support the research of Garrelts et al (1989); Taylor, Hutchison, Milliken, and Larson (1989); Harrigan (1985); and Epperson (1984).

It is recommended that peripheral intermittent intravenous sites be flushed after medication infusions and/or every 8 hours with normal saline solution. As a result of this study and similar findings in other clinical settings, Scott and White Memorial Hospital changed the intermittent intravenous infusion device protocol. Peripheral intermittent infusion devices are now flushed routinely with 1 mL normal saline after drug administration or flushed every 8 hours. (Shoaf and Oliver, 1992)

CONCLUSIONS

The meta-analysis reveals that there is no significant difference between heparin and saline flush procedures in peripheral intravenous catheters. This finding is supported quantitatively by the low average effect size (0.076 ± 0.14) and by the qualitative research data. Results of all but one study suggest that saline solution as a peripheral intravenous flush solution effectively maintains catheter patency, decreases the complications of heparin, and does not significantly increase the incidence of phlebitis. This discrepant study,[5] however, had serious weaknesses. The lack of difference between the two flush solutions is a positive finding in light of the complications associated with heparin use." (Peterson and Kirchoff, 1991)

DISCUSSION

This study supports the findings of others (Epperson, 1984; Garrelts et al, 1989; Hamilton et al 1988) that normal saline is as effective as heparin solution in the maintenance of intermittent peripheral venous access devices. (Geritz, 1992)

6. If the flush solutions compared in the research studies are equally effective in maintaining patency of peripheral locks, how do they compare in cost according to the authors?

Check your answers with those in Appendix A, Chapter 19.

Activity 2

Examine the written protocol on peripheral lock flush procedures that your institution uses. Carefully compare the flush solution and method your institution uses with what was used in the articles in Activity 1.

1. Does your institution use the flush solution that the research in Table 1 reports should be used? Does your institution use the same concentration of solution?

2. What method of flushing the peripheral lock does your institution use? How does the sequence of administering flush solutions compare?

3. How does your patient population compare with the samples in the research studies? Are they older or younger? Is the level of morbidity similar? Does your institution use the same gauge needle as reported in the research studies?

4. If your institution uses a different peripheral lock flush procedure, how much does your procedure cost, and how much would their procedure cost in your institution? Fill in Table 2 to help you with the comparison. If your institution uses the protocol advocated by the research base, fill in the column for your institution only.
   - Cost of solution of heparin? Of saline (single or multi use vials)?
   - Number of times each solution is used?
   - Minutes of staff time required each time the peripheral lock is flushed and average hourly pay (include finding solutions and preparing syringes, as well as administering flush)?
   - Cost of staff time required for each peripheral lock flush?
   - Number of patients in your institution each day that require a peripheral lock?
   - Percentage of patients with a peripheral lock that require flushing the lock?
   - Total number of peripheral lock flushes that are administered in your institution each year?
   - Difference in annual cost of your institution's protocol and that recommended by the research in the three articles?

Check your answers with those in Appendix A, Chapter 19.

Table 2. Comparing the cost of peripheral lock flush protocols

	Saline flush protocol	Your protocol
1. Price of solutions		
a. Saline		
b. Heparin		
2. Number of times each solution is used		
a. Saline		
b. Heparin		
3. Cost of heparin x times used per flush (lines 1a x 2a)		
4. Cost of saline x times used per flush (lines 1b x 2b)		
5. Total cost of solutions (lines 3 + 4)		
6. Minutes of staff time required for flush		
7. Average hourly pay		
8. Average benefit pay (0.18 x line 7 if unsure)		
9. Cost of staff time		
a. Line 7 + line 8		
b. Line 9a divided by 60		
c. Line 9b x line 6		
10. Cost of flush protocol per flush (lines 5 + 9c)		
11. Number of patients that require a peripheral lock		
12. Percent of peripheral locks that are flushed		
13. Total number of peripheral lock flushes (line 11 x line 12)		
14. Annual cost of peripheral lock flush (line 10 x line 13)		

Activity 3

You want to change your institution's protocol on peripheral lock flushes. After a literature search of additional recently published research, you expanded your Summary Table and have identified a strong research base for the change you are proposing. According to the Stetler (1994) model, you have completed Phase II: Validation, and are ready to move into Phase III: Comparative Evaluation. However, you will need to move key people in your institution through Phase II.

1. In your institution, what individuals and disciplines would it be necessary to convince that the practice change has a sufficient research base?

2. How will you convince them to accept the evidence that the practice change has strong research support and is applicable to your clinical setting?

3. If the practice change has comparable patient outcomes to your current practice, how will you demonstrate cost effectiveness, and to whom should you present that evidence?

4. Once the practice change has been approved, how will you or your institution begin the change process?

5. After the practice change has been implemented, is there anything else that must be considered?

Check your answers with those in Appendix A, Chapter 19.

Activity 4

Read the Draucker and Petrovic (1996); Rudy et al (1995); Ward, Berry, and Misiewicz (1996); and Wikblad and Anderson (1995) studies found in Appendix A to D of the textbook.

1. Indicate for each article whether utilization of the results would be conceptual (*C*) or decision driven (*D*):

a. _____ Draucker and Petrovic (1996)

b. _____ Rudy et al (1995)

c. _____ Ward, Berry, and Wisiewicz (1996)

d. _____ Wikblad and Anderson (1995)

2. Think about the implications of each study. Using the questions from Box 19-1 in the text, how important would you consider each study for research utilization in your clinical setting?

   a. What is the topic's priority for nursing and your setting?

   b. What is the magnitude of the problem in your setting? Does it affect a few or many clinical areas? Each study may be considered a priority if the problem addressed is high frequency, high risk, or high cost.

   c. Would the practice change affect length of stay, costs, or patient satisfaction?

   d. For each study, if there were a strong research base, would your setting be ready to change, or are there sensitive issues to consider and address?

3. Is there a research base of other studies on each topic? Look through research indexes to identify other studies on one of the four topics.

Posttest

1. Name four demonstration projects of research utilization:

   a.

   b.

   c.

   d.

2. Match each of the following items to the correct phase of the Stetler (1994) model of research utilization.

   _____ Phase I: Preparation

   _____ Phase II: Validation

   _____ Phase III: Comparative Evaluation

   _____ Phase IV: Decision Making

   _____ Phase V: Translation/Application

   _____ Phase VI: Evaluation

   a. Substantiating evidence

   b. Ongoing CQI/QA

   c. Delay use

   d. Research critique

   e. Specify policy

   f. Study selection

3. List six of the eight elements of essential information to include for each study on a Summary Table:

   a.

   b.

   c.

   d.

   e.

   f.

4. Define the following terms in respect to research utilization:

    a.   Change Champion

    b.   Core Group

    c.   Outcome Data

    d.   Process Data

    e.   Organizational Climate

5. Discuss at least three ways the nurse executive can encourage research utilization.

    a.

    b.

    c.

6. True   False Clinical articles can provide the basis for a practice change.

7. True   False If a research study has any flaws it cannot be used to support a practice change.

8. True   False Cost is as important as clinical outcomes when considering a practice change.

9. True   False Research utilization is an important aspect of the staff nurse role.

The answers to the posttest are in the *Instructor's Resource Manual*.
Please check with your instructor for these answers.

References

Draucker C, Petrovic K: Healing of adult male survivors of childhood sexual abuse, *Image: J Nurs Schol* 28(4):325-330, 1996.

Feldman DL, Rogers A, Karpinski RH: A prospective trial comparing Biobrane, Duoderm and Xeroform for skin graft donor sites, *Surg Gynecol Obstetr* 173:1-5, 1991.

Geritz MA: Saline versus heparin in intermittent infuser patency maintenance . . . including commentary by Hoare K and Jensen L with author response, *West J Nurs Res* 14(2):131-41, 1992.

Hermans MH, Skillman NJ: Clinical benefit of a hydrocolloid dressing in closed surgical wounds, *J ET Nurs* 20(2):68-72, 1993.

Peterson FY, Kirchhoff KT: Analysis of the research about heparinized versus nonheparinized intravascular lines, *Heart Lung* 20:631-42, 1991.

Rudy E et al: Patient outcomes for the chronically critically ill; special care unit versus intensive care unit, *Nurs Res* 44(6):324-331, 1995.

Shoaf J, Oliver S: Efficacy of normal saline injection with and without heparin for maintaining intermittent intravenous site, *Appl Nurs Res* 5(1):9-12, 1992.

Stetler C: Refinement of the Stetler/Marram model for application of research findings to practice, *Nurs Outlook* 42:15-25, 1994.

Ward S, Berry P, Misiewicz H: Concerns about analgesics among patients and family caregivers in a hospice setting, *Res Nurs Health* 19:205-211, 1996.

Wikblad K, Anderson B: A comparison of three wound dressings in patients undergoing heart surgery, *Nurs Res* 44:312-316, 1995.

Appendix A

Answers to Activities

Chapter 1

Activity 1

1. c
2. b
3. d
4. a
5. f
6. e

Activity 2

1. D
2. B
3. C
4. D
5. A
6. B
7. A
8. C
9. B

Activity 3

1. a. DMSc; unknown, head nurse
   b. RN; PhD; RN; MSN
   c. PhD; PhD; PhD; MD; PhD; MSN; RN
   d. PhD; RN; MS; RN; MS; RN
2. a. Yes (*Note:* This author is from Sweden, which uses different initials for degrees than the United States); Yes; Yes; Yes
   b. **Appendix A:** Karin Wikblad, the first author, appears doctorally prepared and could

thus design and conduct the study. No educational preparation is given for the second author, Beth Anderson, but it is mentioned that she is a head nurse, thus she may be a data collector, or even just supportive of having the research conducted on her unit.

Appendix B: Claire Draucker, the first author is a doctorally prepared nurse who has the educational preparation to design and conduct research. The second author, Kathleen Petrovic, is a master's prepared nurse, whose role is not described in the biography.

Appendix C: Authors one (Ellen Rudy), two (Barbara Daly), three (Sara Douglas), and five (Rhayun Song) are doctorally prepared nurses who would obviously be more than qualified to design and implement the study. The fourth author (Hugo Montenegro) is a physician. A medical director of the unit, who developed protocols with the case managers, is mentioned in the article. This may be the medical director, but I am unsure. The sixth author (Mary Ann Dyer) is a master's prepared nurse who is just described as project staff.

Appendix D: Sandra Ward, the first author is doctorally prepared; Patricia Berry, the second author is a doctoral candidate; and the autobiographical statement mentions that the third author, Hollis Misiewicz, is a master's prepared clinician, thus these three authors appear to be appropriate to design and implement a study.

c. **Appendix A:** No mention is made of funding sources in the Wikblad and Anderson article.

Appendix B: The Draucker and Petrovic study was funded by three sources: Delta Xi chapter, Sigma Theta Tau International; the Research Council of Kent State University; and a Biomedical Research Support Grant. Thus, it was subjected to the rigor of three external reviews and deemed valuable enough to be funded by all three.

Appendix C: Rudy et al was funded by a grant from the National Institute of Nursing Research.

Appendix D: The Ward et al study was funded by a NIH Grant to Charles Cleeland, PhD, and the authors thank Professor Cleeland for support of this project. Thus it appears it may have been part of a larger study. However, because there is no mention in the reference list of a published study by Cleeland, it is impossible to know without contacting the authors.

Activity 4

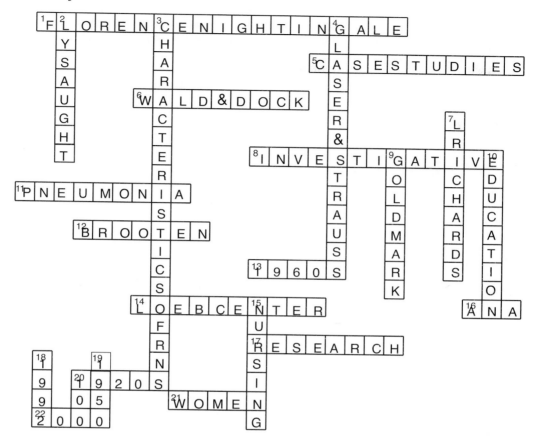

Activity 5

   a.   Continuing to conduct research on the topic of abuse in women
   b.   Developing theoretical perspectives
   c.   Conducting synthesis conferences discussing the area of abuse of women
   d.   Using nursing research studies to assist in legislative change

Activity 6

1.   In order to base my practice on scientific evidence gained through research, I must first understand the research process. Then I need to know how to critique research in order to decide whether particular studies and their results have enough merit to change my practice.
2.   I could share the information with my nurse manager if I worked on an obstetrics floor. However, if I worked in another area, it would still be useful to share these findings with

colleagues in my institution who work in quality improvement or possibly in a discussion group of research findings.

3. Depth in nursing science will occur when a sufficient number of nurse researchers replicate and have consistent findings in a substantive area of inquiry. It is important that each study builds on prior studies, adding new variables or questions as the need arises.

4. Because my area of practice is psychiatric/mental health nursing with an emphasis on chemical dependency, I would like research findings demonstrating that nursing interventions related to "knowledge deficit regarding addiction" have an effect on the outcome of increased sobriety time for the addict or alcoholic.

Chapter 2

Activity 1

1. Rational
2. Active; inner
3. The point of view of the writer
4. Nursing
5. Three (or four)

Activity 2

1. b
2. b
3. a
4. b
5. a
6. a

Activity 3

1. a. Preliminary Understanding
   b. Comprehensive Understanding
   c. Analysis Understanding
   d. Synthesis Understanding
2. a. Read the article for the fourth time
   b. Review your notes on the copy
   c. Summarize study in own words
   d. Complete one handwritten 5 x 8 card per study
   e. Staple the summary to the top of copied article

Activity 4

1. No
2. No
3. Yes (The exact term correlational is not used; however, if you look at the definition of correlation in the glossary, it states that correlation is "the degree of association between the two variables." The authors state the research question as: "(a) What is the strength of association between patient and caregiver concerns?")
4. No (Although the term convenience could be used appropriately to describe this sample.)
5. Yes (The Barriers Questionnaire is the instrument used.) (p. 207)
6. Yes (p. 208)
7. Yes (p. 208)
   Summary: I would categorize this study as quantitative. It meets 5 of the 7 criteria listed. It is not experimental or quasiexperimental (two of the specific types of quantitative that are usually the only designs that would include using the terms hypotheses, control, and treatment group). Instead it is nonexperimental.

Activity 5

I would go to the reference section and locate the articles by Daly et al, which are in *Heart and Lung*, and the Happ article, which is in *Journal of Nursing Administration*. I would then go to the library or an on-line source, find the article and photocopy it or download it for a $12 fee from CINAHL. I would look for the Happ article first, because it appears from the title, *Sociotechnical Systems Theory: Analysis and Application for Nursing Administration*, that this article would contain more information than the other about the theory itself. It is not uncommon to need to seek out primary and secondary sources from the reference list to critically analyze an article.

Chapter 3

Activity 1

1. e
2. b
3. d
4. a
5. c

Activity 2

1. Yes; Yes; Yes; Yes
2. No; No; Yes; Yes
3. Yes; No; Yes; Yes

Activity 3

1. a. CRTs
   b. Birth defects
2. a. Birth defects
   b. Independence/dependence conflicts
3. a. White wine
   b. Serum cholesterol level
4. a. Type of recording
   b. Patient care
5. a. Profession (MD or RN)
   b. Extended-role concept of RNs

Activity 4

1. H_R, DH
2. H_R, DH
3. RQ
4. H_R, DH
5. H_R, NDH
6. RP

Activity 5

1. RQ: Does the use of CRTs by pregnant women influence the incidence of birth defects?
   Ho: The use of CRTs by pregnant women has no effect on the incidence of birth defects.
2. DH: As is in the chapter.
   NDH: There is a difference in the number of independence/dependence conflicts between individuals with and without birth defects.
   H_R: As is.
   RQ: Do individuals with birth defects have a higher incidence of independence/dependence conflicts than those without birth defects?
   Ho: There is no difference in incidence of independence/dependence conflicts between individuals with and without birth defects.
3. DH: There is a positive relationship between daily moderate consumption of white wine and serum cholesterol levels.
   NDH: Daily moderate consumption of white wine influences serum cholesterol levels.
   Hr: There is a relationship between daily moderate consumption of white wine and serum cholesterol levels.
   RQ: As is.
   Ho: There is no relationship between daily moderate consumption of white wine and serum cholesterol levels.

Activity 6

1. a. Yes
    b. Yes; IV-SPID; DV-dressing independence
    c. Yes
    d. Yes
    e. Yes
    f. Yes
    g. Yes
2. a. Yes
    b. Yes
    c. Yes
    d. Yes
    e. Yes
    f. Yes
    g. Yes

Activity 7

a. There is probably not enough time for the student to design and conduct this study. It will take a considerable amount of time to conceptualize this problem and would be a more appropriate study for a doctoral thesis where a student usually has 3 years to resolve a problem. The first year of doctoral study, the student could work on refining the problem in design classes, and then have a full 1 to 2 years to conduct the study, analyze the data, and complete the write-up.
b. This is difficult to answer based on the information given in the brief scenario. Because the nurse has identified it as a problem, I would assume she or he is aware of a unit where this change is occurring; whether the nurse would be able to gain access to that unit to conduct research is an unknown until she or he sends a letter and asks permission of the setting and the setting's Institutional Review Board.
c. The lack of experience of the researcher is probably the greatest impediment to conducting this study. It will take a very experienced and knowledgeable researcher to determine which variables to study and to develop a study design that will give meaningful answers to this question. This is probably why the definitive study in this area has not yet been done.
d. I do not foresee any ethical issues inherent in conducting this study.

Activity 8

The problem statement poses the question the researcher is asking. The hypothesis attempts to answer the question posed by the research problem. The problem statement does not predict a relationship between two or more variables.

Chapter 4

Activity 1

1. Research
2. Education
3. Research; practice
4. Theory

Activity 2

1. f
2. c
3. a
4. e
5. d
6. c
7. b

Activity 3

1. D
2. C
3. D
4. D
5. C
6. D

Activity 4

(*Note:* Choose from any of the following scholarly nursing journals for the five correct answers.) *Advances in Nursing, AORN Journal, Applied Nursing Research, Archives of Psychiatric Nursing, Computers in Nursing, Heart & Lung, Holistic Nursing Practice, Image: Journal of Nursing Scholarship, Journal of Professional Nursing, Journal of Nursing Education, NACOG, Nurse Educator, Nursing Diagnosis, Nursing & Health Care, Nursing Research, Nursing Science Quarterly, Research in Nursing & Health, Scholarly Inquiry for Nursing Practice,* and *Western Journal of Nursing Research.*

Activity 5

1. a. Related Literature
   b. No title given. (*Note:* This is a typical introduction to a qualitative study using grounded theory methodology. In this type of research the researcher will bring some knowledge of the literature to the study but does not usually do an exhaustive search of the litera-

ture. Instead, the researcher allows theory to emerge from the data, a process that will be described in-depth in Chapter 9.)

2. a. Yes, these authors explain that results from prior studies are inconsistent and that further studies are needed to resolve the ambiguities. In their literature review, they do not mention any prior studies specifically of wound dressings after heart surgery or the variables of effectiveness, safety, clinical utility, patient comfort, and cost that I would have expected to be discussed.

   b. Yes, these authors uncover a gap in prior research. They note that although there has been much research on female survivors of childhood sexual abuse, there have been few studies focusing on male survivors.

3. No, the references are very current; they are from 1990 to 1993. It is difficult to write the story from the reference section because there are so few references (i.e., only eight). Two of the articles listed are review articles (Bolton, van Rijswijk, 1991; Cuzzell, 1990). The summary of prior research may be contained in these articles, but it is impossible to know this unless we were to obtain these articles. This literature review does *not* read like a good detective story with one clue or variable after another gradually being eliminated. However, the literature review in a qualitative study would not typically be expected to contain this information, rather it would be expected in the literature review of a quantitative article as described below.

   An example of this process can be seen in the article, Fahs PS, Kinney M: The abdomen, thigh, and arm as sites for subcutaneous sodium heparin injections, *Nurs Res* 40:204-207, 1991 in Appendix A in the 3rd edition of the textbook. It does read like a thorough detective story or a well designed research proposal. The research first cited on the topic is in 1981, where angle of injection, aspiration, and massage of tissue was studied. Then in 1984 three techniques for administering subcutaneous low-dose heparin on formation of bruises was studied. Next in 1988 a study compared two different techniques based on size of syringe and size of air bubble, change of needle, and dry sponge technique. In 1987 the variables of concentration and volume of heparin were studied. Two review articles were written on the topic in 1987 and 1988. Thus when this research was initiated in 1990, new variables were identified to study: the use of alternative sites and bruising.

Activity 6

1. a. S
   b. P
   c. S
   d. S
   e. P
   f. P
   g. P
2. False
3. False
4. True
5. True
6. B, MEDLINE does not contain all nursing references like CINAHL does.

7. True
8. True
9. False

Activity 7

1. D; S
2. D; P
3. D; S
4. D; P
5. D; P

Activity 8

1. What is the source of the material? (*Note:* Look at the last term in the URL address to find the organizational name [it is three letters long]; possibilities include: *com* for commercial organization, *edu* for educational institution, *gov* for government body, *int* for international organization, *mil* for US military, *net* for networking organization, and *org* for anything else. I would feel most comfortable with information gathered from an *edu* or *gov* source, such as www.ncbi.nlm.nih.gov that takes me to the Pub Med Query source for MEDLINE at the US National Library of Medicine [See Appendix B] or from a respected international honor society, such as Sigma Theta Tau International at http://www.stti.iupui.edu/library/.)
2. Is the source a well-respected medical or nursing institution or a federal agency, or is the source an individual putting out his/her own opinion? Critique the source.
3. Is the name of the researcher, or researchers and her/his/their degrees given?
4. Is there a mechanism given to obtain further information about the study or the information presented?
5. Is enough data given in the WEB publication to make a critical analysis about the material, such as the analysis I would make about a research article using the critiquing criteria in the textbook? (*Note:* Remember, in a referred, professional journal usually three independent nursing experts in the field have reviewed the article in a blind review process to determine that this material merits publication.)

Chapter 5

Activity 1

1. Inductive thinking: moves from the particular to the general (or conclusions are developed from specific observations)
   Deductive thinking: moves from the general to the particular (or predictions are developed from known relationships)
2. a. Inductive
   b. Deductive

3. (Observations will vary.)
    If you were able to write a general statement about "headache pain," you used inductive thinking and probably wrote something like:
    X (grimacing) X (rubbing temples) X (grumpy) = indications of headache pain.
    If you were unable to write a general statement, a reason could be that you do not know anyone who has headaches, so you do not have a data base.

Activity 2

1. a. Learned helplessness, self-esteem, depression, health practices, homeless (*Note:* You would also be correct if you listed women.)
    b. Illness uncertainty, stress, coping, emotional well-being, clinical drug trial
    c. Social support, intervention, pregnancy, pregnancy outcome, lower income, African American
    d. Violent behavior, nonviolent behavior, behavior, vulnerable, inner-city youths
    e. Verbal abuse, staff nurses, physicians, stress coping (*Note:* Prevalence and consequences may also be listed as consequences especially if you think of them as capturing an idea.)
2. a. "Beauty" is a concept. "Nursing diagnosis" is a construct.
    b. "Beauty" and "nursing diagnosis" are similar in that both describe an abstraction. Both terms describe some notion that people want to be able to discuss, think about, or use without spending hours describing what is meant.
    c. The terms are different in one important dimension. "Beauty" is a concept that all people recognize, although the precise characteristics of beauty may vary from person to person. The construct, "nursing diagnosis," is an abstraction that has been created by a specific discipline to explain a concept unique to that discipline. All disciplines, especially researchers within a given discipline, create constructs to structure their world of study.
3. There are no "correct" answers for this question. Rather, the thinking that you do to reach a consensus is the "correct answer." An argument could be made for the following as constructs: illness uncertainty, social support intervention, and verbal abuse.
4. a. Answers will vary.
    b. Answers will vary.

Activity 3

1. The two major concepts were surgical wound dressing and clinical aspects. Each of these was operationally defined as follows:
    Surgical wound dressing: One of three types—absorbent, hydrocolloid, or hydroactive. Each dressing was completely defined so that if someone wanted to replicate the study, there would be little problem in duplicating the dressing used.
    Clinical aspects: Clearly defined as effectiveness (wound healing) with clear description of the criteria, safety (i.e., presence of infections and skin changes), clinical utility (i.e., ability to allow ongoing evaluation of the incision), patient comfort (i.e., adhesion, pain at removal), and cost.
2. The concepts of this study were healing and childhood sexual abuse. Given the qualitative nature of this study, precise definitions would not be expected. The intent of this study is to

more clearly articulate the concept.

3. Further explanation for the following terms would be sought: patient outcomes; chronically critically ill; special care unit; and intensive care unit.

Patient outcomes: Defined as length of stay, mortality, readmission to the hospital, complications, patient and family satisfaction, and cost.

Chronically critically ill: Defined by the seven factors listed in Table 1 of this study.

Special care unit: A "seven-bed unit with only private rooms."

Intensive care unit: A "12-bed medical intensive care unit and an 18-bed surgical intensive care unit."

4. The major concepts include concerns, analgesics, patients, family members, and hospice.

Concerns: Defined as responses to items on the Barriers Questionnaire that addresses eight concerns about reporting pain, which are discussed in the article.

Analgesics: This term was not explicitly defined.

Patients: Defined by the four criteria used for inclusion in the study.

Family member: Determined by asking the patient who was most involved in his/her care.

Hospice: Defined as one of two specific agencies.

Activity 4

1. a. 4
   b. 5
   c. 6
   d. 4
   e. 5 or 3
   f. 3
   g. 6
   h. 1
   i. 2
2. a. Wound dressing
   b. i. The characteristics of a good wound dressing are:
      ii. There are complex and important criteria to be used when deciding about wound dressings.
      iii. Advantages of DuoDerm—a wound dressing
      iv. Comparison of different types of wound dressings
      v. Infection rates and costs vary among wound dressings
      vi. Some wound dressings are more comfortable for the client
   c. Deductive
   d. No
   e. None of the above
   f. To find the best wound dressing for clients (evaluated by the five criteria)

Activity 5

CRITIQUING GRID

	Well Done	OK	Needs Help	Not Applicable
1. Theoretical rationale was clearly identified (Could I find it?)	W/A D	R;W/A		
2. The information in the theoretical component matches what the researchers are studying	W/A W/B	D;R		
3. Concepts:				
a. Conceptual definition(s) found	R; W/B	W/A		D
b. Conceptual definition(s) clear	R	W/B		W/A; D
c. Operational definition(s) found	W/A; R	W/B		D
d. Operational definition(s) clear	W/A	R	W/B	D
4. Enough literature was reviewed:				
a. For an expert in the area	R	W/A; D		
b. For a nurse with some knowledge	W/B; R	W/A; D		
c. For a nurse reading outside of area of specialty or interest	W/B; R	W/A; D		
5. Thinking of researcher:				
a. Can be followed through theoretical material to hypotheses or questions	W/A; R	W/B		D
b. Makes sense	W/A; R	D		
6. Relationships among propositions clearly stated	W/A; W/B	R		D
7. Theory:				
a. Borrowed		R		W/A; D; W/B
b. Concepts/data related to nursing	W/B	W/A; D; R		
8. Findings related back to theoretical base. I can find each concept from the theory section discussed in the "Results" section of the report	W/A; W/B R			D

(*Note:* As you see it is not easy to make unequivocal statements about every criterion. Some criteria do not fit one study as well as they fit another study. The use of a grid like the one above is a start in your critical thinking. It makes sure that you have addressed the same areas for each study. You then have to put this information together with your evaluation of the other pieces of the study to make the final critical judgment of the quality of the specific study.)

Chapter 6

Activity 1

1. d
2. c
3. e
4. g
5. h
6. f
7. b
8. a

Activity 2

1. Maturation. The mothers' confidence could be increased by any number of factors, including the act of caring for their infant during the month. The time of measurement could be immediately prior to discharge. Use of a control group would strengthen the findings.
2. Instrumentation. The use of standardized calibrated equipment and training for the volunteers would increase the internal validity of the findings.
3. History. The increase in taxes could account for a decrease in the rate of cigarette smoking. Use of a control group and randomization would improve interpretation of the findings.
4. Selection bias. The differences in smoking cessation rates could be attributed to a number of motivational factors. Random assignment to smoking cessation groups is needed to strengthen this design.
5. Mortality. The program is not successful for single homeless women with preschool children. It is important to look at the make-up of the final study sample when the results are interpreted.
6. Testing. Taking the test repeatedly may be the factor leading to an increase in confidence and accuracy, rather than the experimental program. The use of different outcome instruments and measures may be necessary.

Activity 3

1. a. The setting is a university hospital, presumably in Sweden.
    b. The subjects were 250 patients undergoing elective coronary bypass or valve replacement surgery.
    c. The sample selection criteria is not clearly specified. The report implies that all patients undergoing elective coronary bypass or valve replacement surgery were eligible for the study. This would be a convenience sample. Once selected for the study, the subjects were randomly assigned to research groups.
    d. Sample selection criteria and exclusion criteria were not specified. The use of random assignment into groups and the large sample size help to reduce bias. The report does not describe the similarities or differences among the three groups to help assure the

reader that the groups were similar in composition.

   e.   Yes, the sample was homogenous, consisting of elective coronary bypass and valve replacement surgery patients.

   f.   A series of protocols was used by staff nurses, patients, and public health nurses to measure wound healing, safety related to infection and skin changes, clinical utility, patient comfort, and cost through measurement, rating scales, and self reports.

   g.   Patients assigned to the usual dressing, the conventional absorbent dressing, served as the control group.

Activity 4

1. The design is appropriate to test the research hypothesis. An experimental design is necessary to solve the hypothesis stated as a research objective: to "assess clinical aspects" of wound care products.
2. The researchers use control methods appropriate for experimental research, including random assignment, a control group of usual care, and two experimental groups to test the hypothesis. The variables are measured through strict protocols and standardized instruments.
3. The study is feasible by using a convenience sample and existing staff to help collect the data.
4. The design flows logically from the problem, literature review, and objective (hypothesis implied).
5. Threats to internal validity include any extraneous variables that could influence the results of the study, such as selection bias, mortality, maturation, instrumentation, testing, and history.
6. Internal validity is maintained through reduction of selection bias with random assignment, use of protocols, interrater reliability, training of the nurses, use of raters unaware of experimental conditions.
7. Threats to external validity could include effects of selection, testing, or reactivity.
8. External validity is maintained through randomization and a control group, and use of multiple tests and careful protocols to avoid effects of testing and reactivity. The results are generalizable to other similar patient populations.

Chapter 7

Activity 1

1. Solomon four-group design
2. Time series design
3. After-only experiment
4. After-only nonequivalent control group design
5. True experiment
6. Nonequivalent control group design

Activity 2

1. a. Subjects were randomly assigned to one of three groups by a secretary. The procedure for arriving at the random number was not stated.
   b. The usual absorbent dressing group served as a control group.
   c. There were two experimental dressings to be compared with the usual absorbent dressing. The persons with the hydrocolloid occlusive dressing were in one experimental group and those with the hydroactive dressing were in the other experimental group.
2. Random assignment and use of a control group allow the researcher to observe changes in all three groups. If the assignment is truly random, then potential threats would affect all three groups equally.
3. The study pointed out several factors related to wound dressings and wound healing after surgery. The usual care was found to be better than newer types of dressings for the cardiac surgery patients in terms of safety and cost.
4. Another factor could account for differences. For example, if more older people or persons with other problems were assigned to one of the groups, then another factor could affect wound healing and account for the differences detected.
5. In this instance, the control group treatment of usual care was found to be the best. If the researcher had just compared the two experimental dressings, the study would not have had the same results.

Activity 3

1.

	Pretest	Teaching	Posttest
Group A	X	X	X
Group B		X	X
Group C	X		X
Group D			X

(*Note:* The groups may be arranged in any order, but the four group pattern must be followed.)
2. The nurses would be randomly assigned to each of the groups using a table of random numbers or computer random assignment.
3. The pain knowledge and attitudes questionnaire would be used as a pretest.
4. The teaching program is the experimental treatment.
5. The pain knowledge and attitudes questionnaire is also the posttest or outcome measure.
6. The Solomon four-group design is ideal for experimental studies in which the pretest might affect the outcome. In this case, the questionnaire might change nurses' knowledge and attitudes about pain management. The researcher will be able to compare results for nurses receiving the teaching and not receiving the teaching with and without the pretest.
7. This type of design is particularly effective in ruling out threats to internal validity that the before and after groups may experience. It is effective for highly sensitive issues that might be affected by simply completing a questionnaire as a baseline pretest.
8. A disadvantage of the Solomon four-group design is that a large number of subjects must be available for assignment into the four groups.

Activity 4

1. a. After-only nonequivalent control group design.
   b. Advantages of this design is that the subjects were available for the study. The study is practical and feasible.
   c. Disadvantages include the lack of ability to establish a cause and effect relationship and to generalize the study results to a larger population because of the lack of a randomization.
2. a. True experiment
   b. The advantage of this design is that a cause and effect relationship is clearer in an experimental study in which other factors that could account for the results are controlled through the use of random assignment into treatment and control groups.
   c. The disadvantages of an experimental design include the cost and complexity of strict control measures and the large sample size necessary.
3. a. Quasiexperimental study, nonequivalent control group design.
   b. This design was used because it was not possible to randomly assign subjects to groups. It was possible to conduct pretests and posttests on the groups in order to make comparisons.
   c. The disadvantage of this design is that there are so many factors that account for performance that it is difficult to conclude that the accelerated students have higher performance in other situations. For example, only 27 subjects were in the college graduate group and 29 subjects in the traditional group, which is a fairly small sample for comparison. The groups were demographically similar although the traditional students worked more hours and studied less. Perhaps if the traditional students were also in an accelerated program and worked less the results might be different.
4. a. Time series design
   b. The advantages of this type of design is that it is not possible to use random assignment, but the use of a group similar in characteristics other than irritability allow the researcher to make comparisons. In longitudinal studies each subject can be compared with himself over time to allow trends to be observed.
   c. The disadvantages of this quasiexperimental design is that cause and effect relationships are more difficult to determine when random assignment is not made. The researcher has to carefully examine and compare the groups to determine if another factor accounts for the differences observed.

Activity 5

1. Quasiexperimental designs are usually more practical, more feasible, and more adaptable to real-world practice. In many studies important to nursing, it is not possible to randomize subjects into groups for practical or ethical reasons.
2. The researcher must carefully examine other factors that could account for differences between groups.
3. The clinician must carefully critique the research study and also look for other factors that might explain the results of the study. The results of any study with any design must be evaluated to determine if other factors influence the findings. The results should also be compared with the findings of other similar studies.

Chapter 8

Activity 1

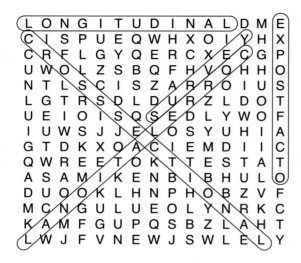

1. Survey
2. Longitudinal
3. Correlational
4. Ex post facto
5. Cross-sectional
6. Correlational
7. Cross-sectional
8. Survey
9. Cross-sectional
10. Cross-sectional

Activity 2

	Advantages	Disadvantages
Correlation studies	A3	D1, D3, D4, D7
Cross-sectional	A1	D2, D5
Descriptive/exploratory	A1	D1, D5
Ex post facto	A4	D1, D2, D3, D4, D5, D7
Longitudinal	A2, A6	D2, D8
Prediction studies	A5	D1
Prospective	A2, A7	D3, D4, D7, D8
Retrospective	A4	D1, D2, D3, D4, D5, D7
Survey	A1	D5, D7

Activity 3

1. M
2. C, D
3. S, CS
4. MA
5. L, S
6. D, R

Activity 4

1. Design-descriptive, exploratory
2. Yes, one of the major points of the text's authors was that consumers must be wary of nonexperimental studies that make causal claims about the findings unless a causal modeling technique is used that was not used in the Mohr study. It appears that the author may have attempted to show a cause-effect relationship among the variables that is not appropriate for an exploratory, nonexperimental study.

Activity 5

Ex post facto

Chapter 9

Activity 1

1. a. Scientific; artistic
   b. Naturalistic settings
   c. Day-to-day living
   d. Lived experience
   e. Smaller
   f. Human uniqueness
   g. Research question
2. a. D
   b. A
   c. C
   d. F
   e. B
   f. I
   g. J
   h. G
   i. E
   j. H

3. Element 1
    a. Study of day-to-day existence for a particular group of individuals
    b. Interested in social processes from perspective of human interactions
    c. Study of the complex cultural aspects related to a phenomenon
    d. An approach for understanding a past event
    Element 2
    a. Query the lived experience, research perspective is bracketed, sample living or has lived the experience
    b. Questions address basic social processes and tend to be action oriented, researcher brings some knowledge of the literature but exhaustive review is not done
    c. Questions are about lifeways or patterns of behavior within a social context, researcher attempts to make sense of world from the insider's point of view
    d. Questions are implicit and embedded in the phenomenon studied, researcher understanding of information without imposing interpretation
    Element 3
    a. Written or oral data may be collected
    b. Collect data through audiotaped and transcribed interviews and skilled observations
    c. Participant observation, immersion, informant interviews
    d. Use of primary and secondary data sources
    Element 4
    a. Move from participant's description to researcher synthesis
    b. Data collection and analysis occur simultaneously, use theoretical sampling, constant comparative method, and axial coding
    c. Data are collected and analyzed simultaneously, searching for symbolic categories
    d. Analyze for importance and then validity (authenticity) and reliability
    Element 5
    a. A narrative elaboration of the lived experience
    b. Descriptive language to show theory connections to the data
    c. Large quantities of data, provide examples from the data and propositions about relationships of phenomena
    d. Well-synthesized chronicle

Activity 2

1. a. Sexual abuse of men has been less frequently studied and less understood than female abuse.
   b. If critical thinking is involved in answering this question, then it is possible that many different ideas may occur to you as ways you might use this information. For example, the review could increase your understanding of male abusers and help you see that victimization may have been experienced earlier in life and could be a root cause for present actions. In thinking about treatment for male assault victims, you might question the adequacy of programs targeted for females as treatment for males.
   c. In critical thinking, there are always more questions to be asked. This literature review provides background understanding for the problem of male abuse. Although some questions about the problem were answered, others were suggested that could have been

included. You will not identify a single right answer, but might think of other topics that could be included. For instance, might attitudes about male victimization in a society that tolerates and perhaps encourages male violence be resistant to seeing treatment as important? Or do men cope differently than women with issues of loss? Other questions might be related to male developmental stages and effects of victimization. Questions such as these might have directed the researchers to include other areas of literature in their review.

Activity 3

1. a. True
    b. False
    c. False
    d. True
    e. True
    f. True
    g. False
    h. True
2. One could identify many ways that knowledge from this study might be applied to nursing practice. The researchers in their conclusion section suggest several applications of this knowledge to practice. For instance, the pervasiveness of problems stemming from occurrences of male abuse victimization might be considered when other health related concerns, such as alcoholism, substance abuse, or domestic violence present as current problems. Counseling related to these issues might include the opportunity to tell stories relevant to childhood experiences and not only focus on current issues. Also, this knowledge could be relevant for the development of practices aimed at primary prevention (Denham, 1995).
3. Replication of studies is costly in the use of resources, and so future studies should build upon existing knowledge. Future studies could aim to develop knowledge more applicable to specific populations. For instance, a study of male sexual abuse that looked at subjects who were incarcerated, gay, or Hispanic would provide more specific knowledge about those populations and enable practitioners increased capability to begin considering generalization to the larger populations.
4. Knowledge about childhood sexual abuse in males may have special relevance for men encountered in your nursing practice. Critical thinking implies looking beyond a solitary right answer and evaluating the usefulness of the knowledge. This includes analysis of the findings in order to consider alternative ways this knowledge might be used, identification of possible consequences, choosing ways to effectively apply what is known, and decide how evaluation will occur.

Activity 4

1. a. D
    b. C
    c. B
    d. A

e. A
f. B
g. C
h. D
i. D
j. A
k. C
l. C
m. D
n. C
o. B
p. A
q. A (could also be true of B or C)
r. A (could also be B, C, or D)
s. C
t. D (could also be true of A or C)
u. C (could also be A)
v. B
w. C

2. a. 3
b. 3
c. 1
d. 4
e. 1

3. This question could have a variety of responses depending upon the qualitative method you select. For instance, in a dissertation study about family health (Denham, 1997), the method selected to study the phenomenon was ethnography. Although other qualitative methods might have been selected to study this phenomenon, ethnography was chosen because it provided the best way to address the research question: How do families define and practice family health in their household settings? The study was designed to better understand gaps in knowledge about the ways families define health, use health information within family context, modify individual health behaviors, and daily practice health within family households. Family and community informants provided audiotaped interviews. Participant observation and journal and field notes were also used as data collection methods. Study subjects were located with the assistance of key informants. The subjects were eight families with a total of 39 family members and 15 community informants. Data analysis initially involved transcription of the interviews and the use of qualitative computer software to sort and categorize the large quantity of data into manageable domains. The analysis included family cases, but constant comparative methods were used to contrast parents, children, and community informant data. Study findings affirmed the importance of family centered health care and the importance of early childhood as a time when health related behaviors were learned. New knowledge pointed to the complex interactions among family and community that create dynamic and evolving patterns of family health and the identification of family health routines as a way to describe individual and family health behaviors.

Chapter 10

Activity 1

1. P
2. N
3. P
4. N
5. N
6. P
7. P

Activity 2

1. b Quota sampling
2. g Systematic sampling
3. d Simple random sampling
4. a Convenience sampling
5. f Cluster sampling
6. c Purposive sampling
7. e Stratified random sampling

Activity 3

1. a. No, the information on the sample was limited to two types of cardiac surgery, gender, age. The report did not include group comparison information other than age.
   b. Partially. Because limited information is given on the sample, the findings may or may not apply to other types of surgical wounds or patients with other factors affecting wound healing.
   c. Nonprobability sample, convenience sample. After selection, the subjects were randomly assigned to treatment groups.
   d. Unsure. The report does not include a power analysis or other information on how the sample size was determined. A large number of variables were measured and compared among three groups; a large sample size is required.
2. One advantage is that it is easy for the researcher to obtain subjects. By limiting the subjects to heart surgery patients at one hospital, the researchers were able to obtain a homogenous sample and control other factors that could confound the study.
3. The disadvantage of a convenience sample is the risk of bias. The researchers used random assignment into treatment groups to reduce bias among groups.

Activity 4

1. True
2. True

3. False
4. False
5. True
6. True

Activity 5

1. The researchers described and compared the subjects in each of the care environments on gender, age, race, prior length of stay, insurance, diagnosis, illness acuity and risks, in addition to stating the eligibility criteria for inclusion in the study.
2. The description of the sample population allows some inferences to be made about the population parameters. The experimental and control group were similar on many parameters. The sample was primarily white. Specific descriptions of factors such as source of payment for care, diagnoses, acuity, and other factors were not given, limiting the ability to draw specific inferences about the population.
3. The sample population represents chronically critically ill patients, but there may be limitations related to ethnicity, socioeconomic factors, or other factors found in other hospital settings. It was not possible to randomly select from all chronically critically ill patients for this study.
4. Eligibility criteria included length of stay, APACHE and TISS criteria, and inability to be cared for on a general nursing unit.
5. Delimitations were included in the eligibility criteria and include no vasopressors, pulmonary artery monitoring, or recent acute event.
6. It would be possible to replicate the study population because the sample population was described with some detail.
7. The sample is one of convenience: all patients in one hospital that met the study criteria were eligible for the study. The method is appropriate because the special care unit was specifically set up for this study.
8. There may be some bias if there is something unique about this particular hospital that may have influenced study results. By using random assignment into treatment groups and careful study protocols, the effects of bias are minimized.
9. There was no information given on sample size requirements, such as a power analysis. The sample is not small and the study received federal funding; presumably a power analysis was conducted. During the discussion the researchers note that "While a significantly lower percentage of SCU patients required readmission, the effect size and power were low, indicating a need for a larger sample size." (Rudy et al, 1995)
10. The procedure includes discussion of the approval by the hospital Institutional Review Board and consent of the primary physician and the patient or next of kin.
11. The researchers discuss limitations and emphasize the need for careful selection of patients for special care units and the need for skilled nurse case managers and collaborative care in alternative settings.
12. Yes, the researchers discuss replication and implications for care in alternative settings.

Chapter 11

Activity 1

1. Nursing Research Committee
2. Justice
3. Expedited review
4. Unethical Research Study
5. Institutional Review Board

Activity 2

1. Respect for persons
2. Beneficence
3. Justice

Activity 3

1. Consent to participate was thoroughly discussed in this article; however, it is important to note that it is done somewhat differently than is typically done in the United States and as described in the text chapter. The authors describe the process under *Procedure*. "When patients arrived on the units, they were signed in by a secretary who presented written information about the voluntary study. A nurse then informed patients orally about the study and offered them the opportunity to participate. After the patient agreed orally to participate, the secretary randomly selected a number from 1 to 3 and put the selected number on the anesthesiologist's order sheet." It is never mentioned that informed *written* consent was obtained. A caveat: typically a nurse researcher or a physician who is capable of explaining the study gives the subject the consent form and answers the subject's questions on-the-spot, however, the secretary gave the patient the initial information sheet in this study.

    In the *Methods* section under *Subjects* of the Wikblad and Anderson (1995) article, the authors state that this study was reviewed and approved by the university hospital Research Ethical Committee. Note: This study took place in Sweden, so they would typically have different titles for committees other than IRB, as is typically used in the United States.

2. In the Draucker and Petrovic (1996) article, the authors state that before the beginning of the interview, participants were asked to read and sign a consent form and to complete a brief demographic sheet. No information is given indicating who presented the form or its contents; however, earlier in the method section the authors state that individuals who had identified themselves as sexual abuse survivors and who had shared their own healing experiences in some public context were contacted individually by the investigators to request their participation. The authors do not indicate whether the other participants were asked to participate by their own service provider or simply asked to contact the investigators, who then explained the study and asked them to participate. The latter would be the preferred method, because it would eliminate any possible feeling of coercion.

    No mention is made in the article of seeking IRB approval. This may be a stylistic consideration of the journal, an editorial decision of the authors, or a matter of space constraints.

3. Consent to participate in the study was covered adequately. Rudy et al (1995) states, "Consent to participate was . . . obtained from both the primary physician and the patient. If the patient was unable to consent, the next of kin was asked for permission; . . . the procedure for consent and group assignment was approved by the hospital's Institutional Review Board" (Rudy et al, 1995). The details of the informed consent were not provided, thus it is not possible to critique the informed consent form or process.

4. **Appendix D:** Informed consent to participate in this study was adequately covered. The authors described the process: "Potential participants were given a letter from the nurse who admitted them to the hospice program inviting them to join the study. Within 24 hours, a data collector telephoned them to discuss their interest and eligibility. If they agreed to participate, the data collector scheduled a home visit within an average of 5 days of their admission to the program. It should be emphasized that the person obtaining the consent and collecting the data was not the nurse providing care. This design decision was based on concern that patients invited by their own nurse might not feel free to decline participation" (Ward, Berry, and Misiewicz, 1996).

    No mention was made of seeking IRB approval.

Activity 4

1. (a-d) Children, elderly, mentally ill, the unborn, persons with AIDS, people in institutions, vulnerable populations (e.g., students or prisoners)
2. The subjects in this study are students. They are a vulnerable population, and therefore, extra precautions must be undertaken to protect their rights.
3. The subjects in this study were adolescents, who make up a vulnerable population, and prisoners, who are both a captive and convenient population, thus extra precautions would need to be taken to guard their rights.

Activity 5

Note: Each student's answer will be different. However, at San Jose State University the composition of the Institutional Review Board: Human Subjects is as follows: one seat designated for a nursing representative, another for a psychology faculty member, a member from Graduate Studies & Research, two student health representatives, a biology representative, a College of Education representative, a Faculty-at-Large member, a Community-at-Large representative, and a student representative. It is informative to note that the programs that have graduate students doing a large number of studies with human subjects such as nursing and psychology have designated seats; also of note is that it is not composed exclusively of faculty but that there is one student and one community member.

Activity 6

(Answers will vary)

1. I had not really thought about this before. I have difficulty with this question because I teach a research course with 75 to 90 students each semester and encourage them to think of

research questions continually; and I would not expect to be acknowledged if a classroom discussion led to a thesis. I believe an acknowledgment would be necessary if the faculty member or clinical mentor spent individual time helping someone to refine a research question or problem.

2. I do not believe so. I am compulsive, as most nurses are, about documentation.
3. Again, this is problematic because of the amount of time and energy that might go into duplicating the material. Although ethically I would feel obligated to share the data, I also believe it would be appropriate to ask for funding for duplicating and any other expenses incurred.

Activity 7

1. One ethical principle guiding research is beneficence; this imparts an obligation to do no harm and maximize possible benefits. Therefore, it would not be ethical to conduct an experimental study at this time. Instead, I would do a descriptive or qualitative study describing the patients and their symptoms and the treatments being used, and then begin to identify all the variables involved.
2. The population of interest is children, who are one of the vulnerable groups; extra precautions must be undertaken to protect their rights. However, at that time there were not guidelines identifying children as a vulnerable population; nor was the Nuremberg Code, which was the original code of ethics for research that was developed after World War II, yet developed. In research involving children, parental consent is required.
3. The study would have to be descriptive, or qualitative, describing in detail all the variables involved.

Chapter 12

Activity 1

Wikblad & Anderson

1. B
2. "Observation is particularly suitable as a data collection method in complex research situations that are best viewed as total entities and that are difficult to measures in parts, . . ." (Gray in Chapter 12). The healing of wounds is a complex entity that requires data from several sources to reach a conclusion but none of the sources can stand alone.
3a. **Nurses' protocol:** (Found at the bottom of page 313 of the study at the bottom of column 2) "Five nurses from each of the three units were trained to examine the dressings. They rated the above parameters for five patients' dressings, compared their ratings that deviated from each other. This procedure was repeated on five new patients until there was total agreement in their ratings."
Level of agreement: Total agreement which equals 100%.
3b. **Photographic protocol:** (found on page 313 toward bottom of column 3) "The evaluation was done by two independent raters, neither of whom was aware of the experimental conditions." The evaluation consisted of rating photographs of the wounds according to redness, degree of healing and skin changes.

Level of agreement: "The kappa coefficient for ratings of wound healing was .81, and the agreement between the two raters was 91%. For ratings of redness, the agreement was 85% (kappa coefficient = .73). To examine intrarater reliability, 5% of the photographs were duplicated. Agreement in those ratings reaching 100%"

3c. **Public health nurses' protocol:** (Found on page 314 at the top of column 1) "During the 4th week after surgery, each patient was asked to have a public health nurse assess the incision and fill in the protocol. The public health nurses' assessment included degree of wound healing (rated on a 3-point scale), redness (yes/no), infection, and treatment with antibiotics (yes/no). Finally, they were asked to describe the skin around the incision. Once completed, the protocols were mailed to the clinic."

Level of agreement: Not reported.

Draucker and Petrovic

1. C
2. A
3. Geographic constraints
4. The basic rationale for using interviews was the desire to collect a great quantity of very rich and complex data in an area that had not been previously studied.

Rudy et al

1. E
2. D
3. The predominant use of records with guided evaluative procedures was used to assess the world as it existed. Was interested in reaching a conclusion given available information. Would have also been more cost efficient.
4. Nurses were trained in the use of the instruments with reliability checks completed at each point. A summary paragraph is found on page 327 of the study about midway in the second column. It begins: "Since each instrument is dependent upon accurate abstraction data from the patient record, interrater agreement was carefully monitored." The authors then proceed to explain how this occurred.

Ward, Berry, and Misiewicz

1. D
2. B
3. 1. I would have some concern about the vocabulary level of the Barriers Questionnaire. If the vocabulary used in Table 2 reflects the words actually used in the questionnaire, an assessment of reading skill would have been appropriate.
   2. I need more information about the consistency among subjects regarding pain experience. If the pain experience of breast cancer is comparable to that of pancreatic cancer, then data may be comparable. Does the "admitted to hospice within 48 hours" control this factor?
   3. The internal consistency measures raised some thoughts about the degree of faith I could have regarding some of the subscales.

Activity 2

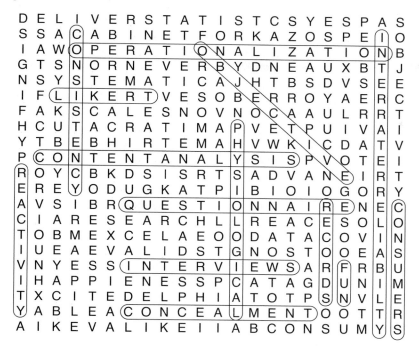

1. Consumers
2. Physiological
3. Reactivity
4. Interviews
5. Records
6. Questionnaires
7. Objectivity, consistency
8. Concealment
9. Interrater reliability
10. Operationalization
11. Likert scale
12. Fun

Activity 3

1. If I were wanting to observe the influence of different testing skills on the behavior of preschoolers being given a cognitive skill based instrument, I would consider using a one-way window.
2. I would obtain consent from the parents of the children and the agency in which the testing would be performed.
3. Concealment with intervention.

Activity 4

Physiological measures would be of minimal use since the data I am seeking would not involve actual measures of the residents' physiological status. Not particularly interested in current blood pressure, temperature, urinary output, etc.

Could consider using observation, e.g. sitting in an emergency room and observing the types of health care concerns that enter. Would need to think about whether or not this would be observation with concealment. Would need to wrestle with the notion of what is private information and what is public domain information.

Could use questionnaires and collect data from all types of health care providers. Could give me a lot of data in a short time. Wonder how busy they would be and what would be the probability of their filling out the questionnarie?

Could use an interview. Is costly in terms of researcher time, but could get me the information in more detail because I could ask them to expand upon specific items. But who would I want to interview? How do I get into their offices/homes, etc?

Need to get some information from the people who actually live here. Wonder how I could reach a cross section of those individuals? Could I call? What about those people without a telephone?

Better check out the census data to get a clearer picture of what I am dealing with. Probably have some morbidity and mortality data collected by the state health department. I would probably utilize existing records to get a first sense of what the parameters of "health" are in this community. Then I would talk to some people about who knew the most about this area and arrange some interviews with these individuals. These would be guided interviews with open ended items to encourage the sharing of as much information as possible. I would also seek a way to collect data from a variety of health care users, e.g. surveys in the waiting room of various agencies, maybe the crowd at a mall, at a county fair.

One data collection instrument would not be sufficient to collect the information needed about the areas addressed.

Activity 5

1. D
2. A
3. D
4. A, B, C
5. D

Chapter 13

Activity 1

1. S; avoided by proper calibration of the scale.
2. S; decrease error by providing instructions, ensuring confidentiality, or other means to allow

students to freely express themselves.

3. R; lessen by training research assistants and using strict protocols or rule books to guide analysis.

4. R; decrease their anxiety by addressing their concerns, providing comfort measures or other efforts that might decrease their anxiety. Anxiety may alter the test responses.

Activity 2

1. Content; criterion-related; construct
2. Rating from a panel of experts
3. Criterion-related or concurrent
4. Construct
5. Multitrait-multimethod
6. Face
7. Hypothesis testing; factor analysis; convergent and divergent approaches; contrasted-groups
8. Convergent; divergent

Activity 3

1. Stability; homogeneity; equivalence
2. Test-retest methods could be accomplished by giving the same test again at a later date and seeing if the two scores are highly correlated. Parallel or alternate forms, such as alternate versions of the same test, could also be used to establish stability.
3. Alternate forms would be better if the test taker is likely to remember and be influenced by the items or the answers from the first test.
4. a. 2
    b. 4
    c. 1
    d. 3
5. Interrater reliability

Activity 4

1. Yes
2. Yes
3. Factor analysis and comparison of the factors to the original work
4. Yes (*Note:* Statistically tested to be the same)
5. Yes
6. Yes (*Note:* Briefly in the results section, they comment that satisfaction scores tended to be high and did not vary. Use of this tool was discontinued because it did not provide useful information for the continuation of the study. Satisfaction was high for both groups.
7. Members of the research team were trained and monitored to achieve at least 90% agreement before they independently collected data. They also conducted periodic interrater reliability checks and updated coding rules.

Chapter 14

Activity 1

1. d
2. c
3. d
4. a
5. a, b, or c
6. a
7. b
8. d
9. a
10. c

Activity 2

1. a. Mood state; ordinal or interval (*Note:* The researchers treated the data as interval based on some characteristics of the data. It is not uncommon for data collected with a Likert scale to be treated as interval. You must determine for yourself the degree of faith you have in the ability to measure the quantity of difference between categories of agreement with a particular statement.)
   b. Perceived health status; nominal
   c. Abuse status; nominal
   d. Calories; ratio
   e. Mother's age; trimester of contact, and birthweight; age at ratio level, *trimester at nominal, birthweight at ratio
   *The interval level of measurement would also be considered a correct answer. It depends on whether an age of 0 can be conceptualized and how conservative the statistician is.
2. a. Mood state; only the first line
   b. Mean; standard deviation; study range; and possible ranges
   c. Interval or ratio
   d. Yes
   e. Yes, data were at the nominal level of measurement and simple percentages were calculated. The women would have answered "yes" or "no," thereby placing them in a category. The number of people in the "yes" category was used to calculate the percentage of the total sample.
   f. Abused women were more likely to enter prenatal care during the third trimester than nonabused women.
      There are ethnic differences in the number of women abused within the past year.
      There are ethnic differences in the percentage of low-birth-weight babies.
   g. Yes, means and standard deviations are used with interval or ratio data. Calories are measured at the ratio level.

h. The mean number of calories consumed daily for the 78 adolescent males was 3,322. The lowest number of daily calories consumed was 435; the greatest number of calories consumed was 7,753. If it is assumed that the distribution of calories consumed fits a normal distribution, then 68% of the subjects consumed between 2,059 and 4,585 calories daily.

Activity 3

Across

1. Goofy's best friend
3. Old abbreviation for mean
5. Abbreviation for number of measures in a given data set (the measures may be individual people or some smaller piece of data like blood pressure readings)
8. Describes a set of data with a standard deviation of 3 when compared with a set of data with a standard deviation of 12
10. Abbreviation for standard deviation
11. Marks the "score" where 50% of the scores are higher and 50% are lower
12. Measure of variation that shows the lowest and highest number in a data set

Down

1. The values that occur most frequently in a data set
2. 68% of the values in a normal distribution fall between ±1 of this statistic
4. Can describe the height of a distribution
6. Describes a distribution characterized by a tail
7. Very unstable
9. Measure of central tendency used with interval of ratio data

Activity 4

1. 142.63
2. a. Wives
   b. Total problem score
3. The wives' score in "Self Ability" of "Marital Empathy" (i.e., SD = 6.32)
4. Husbands
5. Yes, the table and narrative agree.

Activity 5

1. a. Yes
   b. No
   c. Yes
   d. Yes
2. a. Yes
   b. No
   c. Yes

     d. Yes
3. a. Demographic characteristics of sample, wound healing
     b. N/A
     c. Demographic characteristics of sample, basic data on patient outcomes
     d. Demographic characteristics of sample, data regarding "concerns"
4. a. Yes
     b. N/A
     c. Yes
     d. Yes
5. Ward, Berry, and Misiewicz

Chapter 15

Activity 1

Answers found in *Instructor's Resource Manual*.

Activity 2

There are no answers for this activity. Check with your instructor if you have specific questions about the use of the statistical techniques in any of these studies. Most of the studies are fairly complex. They are listed so you can look through them and get a sense of how inferential techniques are used and presented in actual studies.

Activity 3

1. Is there any difference among the three types of dressings?
2. Implied
3. There will be a difference among the three types of dressings in terms of effectiveness, safety, clinical utility, comfort, and cost. (*Note:* To be precise, each set of variables would be written as a separate hypothesis so that there would be a minimum of five hypotheses in this study.)
4. There will be no difference among the three types of dressings in terms of effectiveness, safety, clinical utility, comfort, and cost.
5. The null hypothesis is the one that can be tested through the use of mathematical (i.e., statistical) formulas. One cannot prove the existence of a difference; rather, one can only find "no support" for the fact that no difference exists. The best I can do as a researcher is state: "Based on the evidence in this study, it would be exceedingly rare (or highly improbable) that results this weird would have happended by chance. With results this strange (and because I trust my research design, sampling strategies, and data collection methods), I am going to infer that the independent variable created the odd results."

6. Independent Variable(s):   Type of dressing
   Dependent Variable(s):   Effectiveness (wound healing)
                            Safety (presence of infections and skin changes)
                            Clinical utility (ability to allow ongoing evaluation of incision)
                            Patient comfort (adhesion, pain at removal)
                            Cost
7. Differences among groups
8. There are three categories of the independent variable. Each category is a different type of dressing: hydroactive, hydrocolloid, and conventional.
9. Wound healing = nominal
   Safety = frequency of specific microbes that can be labeled as nominal
   Clinical utility = nominal
   Patient comfort = nominal
   Cost = nominal was the basis in terms of counting the number of dressings that were then multiplied by the cost
10. Chi-square
11. Yes
12. I would choose the conventional absorbent dressing. The degree of discomfort was greater with the other two dressings. The chi-square was statistically significant in both comparisons, so I would infer that the difference in pain was due to something other than chance. This type of dressing is the most likely candidate.
13. *Note:* This could have been tricky. Check your answer before you go any further. Does it discuss clinical significance and not statistical significance?

    Type I error is the rejection of the null hypothesis when it is really true. Now think about the "pain at removal" data. The tested null hypothesis would be that "there is no difference in pain when any of the three dressings is removed." The researchers rejected this statement, which implies that there is a difference among the dressings. If a Type I error was committed, it meant the null should have been supported, that is, there is no difference. It makes no difference which dressing is chosen because the patient's pain will be the same when the dressing is removed.

Activity 4

1. Establishing the "preexperimantal" equivalencies of groups minimizes the criticism that the result or outcomes of the study could have been attributed to differences that were present in the groups before the intervention was implemented. The patients in ICU could have been more critically ill, which would have been a competing explanation for the findings. Establishing that acuity of illness was equivalent in both groups addresses this competing explanation.
2. "Readmit" outcome
3. The data for this outcome were collected using categorical measures.
4. a. Transportation and other financial problems
   b. Health care providers need to pay attention to these factors, especially in mothers at risk for LBW infants.
5. a. Hopelessness and health-related hardiness = -0.63

Hopelessness and uncertainty = 0.46

    b. As the scores on hopelessness increased (i.e., as one became less hopeful), the scores on health-related hardiness decreased. Hopelessness and uncertainty moved together as one (i.e., as one increased, the other increased, too).

    c. No specific answer for this item.

6. "Stepwise multiple regression" was used to examine the predictability of adjustment using the study variables in Table 3. Hopelessness and income were significant predictors of adjustment. More than 38% of adjustment's variance was determined by the variable of hopelessness, although income accounted for an additional 14% of the variability. No other variable contributed to the regression model at the 0.05 significance level.

7. The Time I (pretransplant) values for QLI, HF, and PS in relation to the other posttransplant times of measurement.

Chapter 16

Activity 1

1. a. A
    b. B
    c. B
    d. B
    e. A
    f. A
    g. A
    h. B
    i. B
    j. B

2. a. False
    b. True
    c. True
    d. False
    e. True

3. The absorbent dressing promotes better wound healing, is less costly, easier to remove, and less painful for the patient when it is removed. The hydroactive dressing is the least preferred dressing based on the variables examined. The hydrocolloid dressing may be considered as an alternative to the absorbent dressing although it is more costly and more painful for the patient when removed.

4. a. The hydroactive dressing group had significantly more wounds with excessive redness than the absorbent dressing group (48% to 16% respectively).

    b. There is no statistically significant difference in the number of wounds with redness between the two groups.

    c. 1. C
        2. B

3. A
4. E
5. D

d. True

e. True

Activity 2

1. Surviving childhood sexual abuse is like escaping a dungeon and becoming free. It consists of four phases: (1) living in the dungeon, (2) breaking free, (3) living free, and (4) freeing those left behind. Feelings of entrapment, abandonment, disconnectedness, quitting, and abnormality prevail. Freedom develops by breaking free from the psychological labels self-imposed and awakening a healthy sense of self-achieving normalcy.

2. a. Nurses should realize the childhood sexual abuse experience can be pervasive and deeply disturbing for the male survivors.
   b. Nurses should thoroughly assess the depth and breadth of the clients' recollections of the sexual abuse experience.
   c. Nurses must understand these types of clients feel diseased, abnormal, and alien-like.
   d. Male survivors need help to break free from the psychological dungeon they live in, and it will involve a tremendous amount of time and effort.
   e. Nurses must realize that breaking free also involves overcoming a societal stigma attached to the experience.

3. a. Replicate the study with female survivors.
   b. Compare survivors from various socioeconomic levels.
   c. Write testable hypotheses using the theoretical framework developed by the researchers.

Activity 3

1. a. Patients; Caregiver
   b. 4
   c. 2
   d. The majority of subjects for both groups are married, with a minimum of a high-school education, and make less than $29,000/year.

2. a. 2
   b. 4
   c. False
   d. Caregiver and patients do not share the same concerns about reporting pain and using analgesics.

3. a. False
   b. 2
   c. The findings are inconsistent. There appears to be no statistically significant difference between the patient and caregiver regarding concerns about reporting and using analgesics. This does not presume they are in agreement. Further research in this area is indicated.

4. a. Patients and caregiver do not differ or correlate on their concerns about reporting pain and using analgesics. The results are inconsistent.
    b. Nurses need to further investigate the concerns of both the patient and the caregiver with respect to reporting and using analgesics. Individual concerns must also be addressed.
    c. Several limitations of the study may have influenced the results, such as homogeneity of the sample, small sample size, characteristics of the sample, data collection procedures, and the amount of missing data. Replication is strongly suggested.
    d. Nurses should study patients and caregiver over time to identify an adequate protocol for managing patient's pain.
    e. Nurses should thoroughly assess the pain management needs of hospice patients in order to help the patient and caregiver through the terminal life stages.

Activity 4

1. The purpose of the study is to compare the effects of a low-technology environment of care based on a nurse-managed care delivery system (SCU) with the traditional high-technology (ICU) environment based on primary nursing care delivery system.
2. a. Length of stay
    b. Mortality
    c. Readmission to the hospital
    d. Complications
    e. Patient and Family Satisfaction
    f. Cost
3. ANOVA (Analysis of variance); Chi-square
4. 4
5. 4
6. * Chronically ill patients can safely be cared for in the SCU.
    * There is no statistically significant difference between ICU and SCU regarding mortality rates, length of stay, readmission rates, complications, and patient/family satisfaction.
    * Cost is a major difference between the two units. ICU is much more costly for the patient.
    * Carefully selected chronically ill patients can be transferred to the SCU with no threat to patient safety and with considerable cost savings to patients.
    * As the ICU nurse manager, you would develop a protocol for determining when a patient could be transferred to the SCU.

Chapter 17

Activity 1

Problem Statement and Purpose

1. "The objective of the present study was to assess clinical aspects of a semiocclusive hydroactive dressing and an occlusive hydrocolloid dressing in comparison with a conven-

tional absorbent nonocclusive wound dressing."

2. Yes—not variables per se but the idea is clear that "type of dressing" will be evaluated in terms of "clinical aspects." "Type of dressing" would be considered the independent variable and "clinical aspects" would be the dependent variable.

3. The purpose does not state the population, but the very first sentence of the article indicates that the focus will be individuals who had heart surgery.

4. The significance of the problem was identified in the first paragraph of the article.

Review of Literature and Theoretical Framework

1. The literature review addresses the clinical reports of use of the different dressings. The results of each of these various studies are related to the clinical "effectiveness" characteristics identified by the authors as important.

2. This study is placed in the context of previous literature. There is no theoretical framework that is appropriate in a study of this type.

3. Conflicts among previous works and less than the desired level of information are noted. See the last sentence of the *Related Literature* section.

4. All are primary sources. Reference list does include a statistical method resource.

5. Operational definitions are alluded to at the end of the introductory paragraphs. Greater detail regarding most of the clinical outcomes was provided in the methodology section of the report. "Adhesion" was addressed only tangentially.

Hypotheses or Research Questions

1. There were no hypotheses stated. No specific research question was stated in question format; nevertheless, the question to be addressed was clear.

2. N/A

3. N/A

4. N/A

5. N/A

6. N/A

Sample

1. No specific selection was mentioned and the use of only one facility was discussed; therefore, it is assumed that the sample was one of convenience.

2. The procedures that were used were clearly discussed. There was no use of a tightly structured sampling methodology. Clients were assigned to the treatment groups randomly.

3. Two questions need to be considered when thinking about generalizability: (1) how closely do the sample demographics match comparable clients in my facility? and (2) how great is the chance that dressing change procedures would be so different between agencies (in different countries) that different results would be possible?

4. Yes

Research Design

1. Quasiexperimental

2. None given

3. Yes

Internal Validity

1. *History* did not present a problem as far as we know. No special event occurred during the running of the study that would have broadly influenced the results. *Maturation* was controlled by the researchers (see *Procedures*). *Testing* was not a factor as there were no pretest

or posttest conditions. *Instrumentation* was addressed by training the observers before the data collection. *Mortality* was addressed. Drop-outs were addressed with an explanation given for their not being included in the final set of data. Explanations were valid and 78% of the original group did provide adequate data. *Selection bias* was addressed by randomly assigning clients to each of the three dressing groups.

External validity

1. One would want to exercise caution in considering the representativeness of the sample. This is not to say that the sample is not representative (it would just need to be a point to consider before generalizing) but is there any systematic difference between Swedish patients and US patients?

Methods

1. Observation; wound culture; self-report
2. Yes

Legal-Ethical Issues

1. Is not specified. It was mentioned that the study had been "reviewed and approved by the university hospital Research Ethical Committee" and that would lead one to think that adequate safeguards were in place.
2. Is explained in the first paragraph of the *Procedure* section

Instruments

1. N/A
2a. Nurses were specified as the observers in most instances. Nurses were not specifically mentioned as the individuals who evaluated photographs of the wounds. One would think they would have been nurses. If not, could be a limitation.
2b. Training method was made explicit and was appropriate.
2c. The protocols mentioned in the study served as observational guides.
2d. Yes
2e. No
3-5. N/A

Reliability and Validity

1. Reliability was discussed in terms of the nurse observers being trained until they were in total agreement. Interrater reliability was addressed in the discussion of the evaluation of the photographs.
2. Observers = total agreement
   Photograph evaluators = 91%, 85%, 100% that are all acceptable
3. Validity required is that of face validity—yes the methods were valid for collecting the type of information that was collected. Appropriate safeguards were in place.

Analysis of Data

1. Nominal
2. Descriptive and inferential
3. Yes (nominal data and use of chi-square)
4. Yes
5. Actual probabilities are reported rather than the *a priori* setting of an acceptable level of alpha.
6. No tables or figures were used.

Conclusions, Implications, and Recommendations

1. N/A
2. Yes
3. No specific limitations were addressed
4. Several were mentioned: client comfort, healing, cost were the main ones.
5. Conventional dressing appears to be the best for heart surgery incisions.
6. Perhaps a bit—this is where one's own clinical expertise becomes a factor. This is not my area of expertise (I have not been involved with heart surgeries for several years, and I do not know the literature). It is possible that the extent of the literature is such that this study can sit as the definitive one in a chain of studies or there may need to be some additional work. This is a judgment call.
7. None

Chapter 18

Activity 1

1. Each theme has several examples of data that support the selection of the term. You may have selected a different example.
   a. "The expression in stone and mortar of the power and hatred of the builders"
   b. "Having problems snowball on top of me"
   c. "Shut up, you're a man, you're not supposed to cry"
   d. "Deadening" of feelings
   e. Deprived of being able to fully participate in the activities of everyday life

Activity 2

1. You may have thought of many different factors. An example of something you might consider when deciding whether these findings are applicable is the degree of similarity between the original study and the new group of interest. If there is much similarity in subject demographic characteristics then the findings might be fitting to apply. An important factor to always consider when applying qualitative findings is that individuals are unique. Findings that may be applicable to groups may not necessarily be characteristic of specific individuals.
2. Context bound means findings from qualitative studies that describe specific processes or particular phenomena that should be viewed from a contextual perspective. This context may have cultural, historical, traditional values and mores tied to time and place that are specific to the population studied.
3. The men in this study were all sexually abused as children, but the actual characteristics of the context surrounding the victimizations differed. The research report does not describe the ages of the men when the sexual abuse occurred, but mentions that the duration of the experience ranged from a single incident to many years and that the perpetrators were mostly acquaintances. Replication of this study could be more context bound by including only males who were repeatedly abused by acquaintances. By narrowing the selection factors for

the subject, although the findings would still not be generalizable, greater group homogeneity increases the contextual commonality.

4. Sexual abuse of males
5. The findings could aid in the development of an instrument to investigate the pervasive effects of childhood abuse experiences on male survivors.

Activity 3

1. a. G
   b. B
   c. D
   d. A
   e. F
   f. D
   g. E
   h. G
   i. B
2. a. The researchers' conclusions that emotional pain and societal expectations that men should not be victims appear as plausible reasons why male children might keep their feelings locked inside and feel as if they lived in a dungeon.
   b. The researchers provided data within the report that supported each theme identified as findings. Although I might have questions about some areas, I know that the writing of a research report for a journal is restricted in page length and limits the researchers' ability to tell everything that might be supportive. This issue can be especially problematic to qualitative researchers who often have large quantities of data in the form of transcribed interviews. If more information was desired it would be appropriate to contact the researchers.
   c. The detail in the thematic discussion of the findings gave much support to the researchers' interpretations of living in the dungeon, breaking free, living free, and freeing those left behind. The data from the study participants appeared to fit with the thematic interpretations made by the researcher and seemed to be ideas that had relevance for nursing practice.

Activity 4

Several areas of concern might be identified and there are not necessarily singular answers that are right or wrong. Three examples are provided as a way to consider the value of the knowledge generated by the study; two concerns are related to the study participants and one is related to data collection.

First, the 20 years since the war may have affected the perceptions these nurses had about their experience and their responses may have been very different from what might have been expressed more immediately following their return from Vietnam.

Second, the fact that the majority of these nurses volunteered might make this population of nurses very different from a population that may not have had a choice. For instance, in more recent times, nurses in the National Guard were called up and given orders to leave for Desert

Storm within a week with little time to prepare for the experience. This experience might have been a very different war experience than one where nurses who volunteered had the opportunity to consider the decision and make a choice. Different populations might identify different meanings of nursing wartime experiences.

A third concern is related to the questions asked during data collection. Other questions may have provided different knowledge and perhaps have been more important in understanding nursing during war including questions such as: (1) What were the difficult things you encountered as you practiced nursing during a wartime setting?, (2) What essences of nursing seemed different when experienced during a war? and (3) What ways do you think doing wartime nursing affected your nursing career and practice? Because the majority of these nurses responded so long after the war experience, questions such as these might have built greater knowledge about ways nursing during a war experience affected later nursing practice.

Critique of a qualitative study allows the persons evaluating the work to consider what might have been learned had the study been designed differently and compare the current findings with the value of what might have been learned using alternative methods. Critique does not necessarily mean what was done or discovered was wrong, but allows the chance to view alternative methods for future research, think about what the investigator really wants to learn given the limitations of the study, think about the generalizability of the findings, and evaluate the knowledge learned.

Chapter 19

Activity 1

1. Yes
2. Geritz (1992) examined 150 peripheral IV lock sites, Shoaf and Oliver examined 260 adult surgical subjects, and Peterson and Kirchhoff (1991) included 20 studies in a meta-analysis. Of those 20 studies, 19 focused on adult subjects. The patients are relatively comparable, although Geritz (1992) has a small sample size.
3. All three studies are comparing similar flush protocols.
4. All three studies concluded there was no difference in patency or phlebitis when comparing the flushing protocols.
5. Geritz addressed the cost issue in the discussion and recommended the use of saline only as a flush solution. The other two studies addressed cost in the introduction and recommended the saline flush protocol in the conclusions. Peterson and Kirchhoff did not explicitly consider the cost of nursing time.
6. All three studies indicate a saline flush protocol is lower in cost than a heparin flush protocol.

Activity 2

1. Answer will vary by clinical setting.
2. Answer will vary by clinical setting.
3. Answer will vary by clinical setting.
4.

Comparing the cost of peripheral lock flush protocols

	Saline flush protocol*	Your protocol*
1. Price of solutions		
a. Saline	$0.10	$0.10
b. Heparin	$0.45	$0.45
2. Number of times each solution is used		
a. Saline	1	1
b. Heparin	0	1
3. Cost of heparin x times used per flush (lines 1a x 2a)	$0.10	$0.10
4. Cost of saline x times used per flush (lines 1b x 2b)	$0.00	$0.45
5. Total cost of solutions (lines 3 + 4)	$0.10	$0.55
6. Minutes of staff time required for flush	7	10
7. Average hourly pay	$13.00	$13.00
8. Average benefit pay (0.18 x line 7 if unsure)	$2.34	$2.34
9. Cost of staff time		
a. Line 7 + line 8	$15.34	$15.34
b. Line 9a divided by 60	$0.26	$0.26
c. Line 9b x line 6	$1.79	$2.56
10. Cost of flush protocol per flush (lines 5 + 9c)	$1.89	$3.11
11. Number of patients that require a peripheral lock	200	200
12. Percent of peripheral locks that are flushed	0.50	0.50
13. Total number of peripheral lock flushes (line 11 x line 12)	100	100
14. Annual cost of peripheral lock flush (line 10 x line 13)	$68,972.83	$113,393.33

* These costs are an example of the calculations and will vary by clinical setting.

The difference in cost would be the difference between your institution's protocol and the saline flush protocol line 14 of Table 2.

Activity 3

1. At many institutions a physician must order the flush solution for IVs. Pharmacy may also be involved in stocking, labeling, and preparing flush solutions. Therefore, it would be beneficial to include representatives from Nursing, Medicine, and Pharmacy. Different departments may request including their own representatives in any discussions of this practice change. Having department heads or other people in power positions appoint representatives

rather than depending on volunteers will add value to your endeavor.

2. Some representatives will accept your information at face value. However, to prevent any opposition from the beginning, it may be advisable to prepare the Summary Table, and distribute it and copies of the articles as well.

3. In this example, cost effectiveness may be demonstrated by calculating supplies and staff time cost. However, an intervention may initially cost more in time and supplies, yet cost less overall due to improved clinical outcomes.

4. It is important to proceed through the appropriate channels for your institution. Policies and procedures should be written to reflect the practice change. Communication to all departments affected is essential, possibly both in writing and presentation at departmental meetings. Sometimes the communication may be through the departmental representatives who were appointed earlier. Education for all staff affected should be thorough and include all shifts and units. Concise written information should be available on the practice change in areas that staff frequent. Individual unit representatives could be educated in depth, and would then be available on the unit for questions and education.

5. After implementation of the practice change, it is important to assess compliance with the practice change and watch for potential adverse events. What are patency and phlebitis rates for saline flush only when compared with rates prior to the change in flush solutions?

Activity 4

1. a. C
    b. D
    c. C
    d. D
2. a-d. Answers will vary by clinical setting.
3. Answers will vary by topic identified. See example on CD-Rom in Chapter 4, the Web exercise where a search was done for articles related to the Wikbland and Anderson study (1995).

Please proceed to the enclosed CD-Rom for additional activities.

Appendix B

Home Pages

Agency for Health Care Policy and Research

US Government site that provides links to research portfolio, guidelines, and medical outcomes, consumer health information, news, and resources, and electronic catalog.

URL: *http://www.ahcpr.gov/*

National Library of Medicine–PubMed

Provides free access to MEDLINE's search service to access 9 million citations. Searches by terms, authors, or journal titles. Provides sets of related articles pre-computed for each article cited.

URL: *http://www.ncbi.nlm.nih.gov/PubMed/*

Virginia Henderson International Nursing Library

Sigma Theta Tau International's Honor Society of Nursing web site which has links to the Registry of Nursing Research (free to members as of 1/98) and The Online Journal of Knowledge Synthesis (provides a critical review of research pertinent to clinical practice problems) available with a subscription fee.

URL: *http://www.stti.iupui.edu/library/*

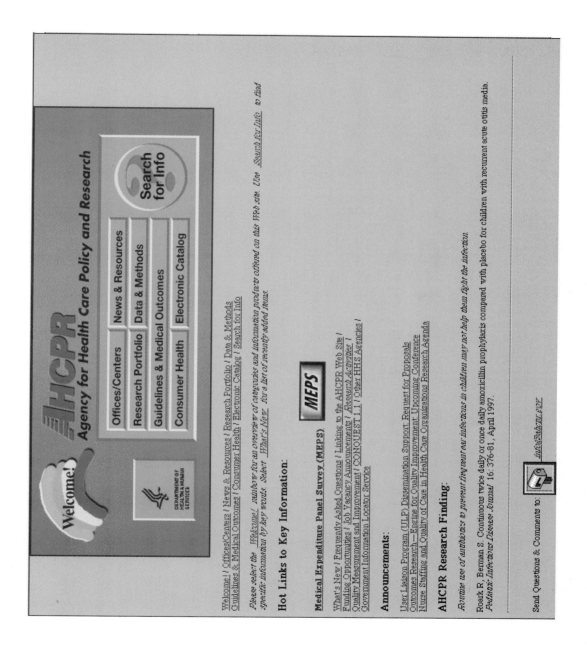

Welcome! / Offices/Centers / News & Resources / Research Portfolio / Data & Methods
Guidelines & Medical Outcomes / Consumer Health / Electronic Catalog / Search for Info

Please select the Welcome! rainbow for an overview of resources and information products offered on this Web site. Use Search for Info to find specific information by key words. Select What's New for a list of recently added items.

Hot Links to Key Information:

Medical Expenditure Panel Survey (MEPS)

What's New / Frequently Asked Questions / Linking to the AHCPR Web Site /
Funding Opportunities / Job Vacancy Announcements / Research Activities /
Quality Measurement and Improvement / CONQUEST 1.1 / Other HHS Agencies /
Government Information Locator Service

Announcements:

User Liaison Program (ULP) Dissemination Support: Request for Proposals
Outcomes Research—Engine for Quality Improvement: Upcoming Conference
Nurse Staffing and Quality of Care in Health Care Organizations: Research Agenda

AHCPR Research Finding:

Routine use of antibiotics to prevent frequent ear infections in children may not help them fight the infection.

Roark, R; Berman S. Continuous twice daily or once daily amoxicillin prophylaxis compared with placebo for children with recurrent acute otitis media. *Pediatric Infectious Disease Journal* 16: 376–81, April 1997.

Send Questions & Comments to: *info@ahcpr.gov*

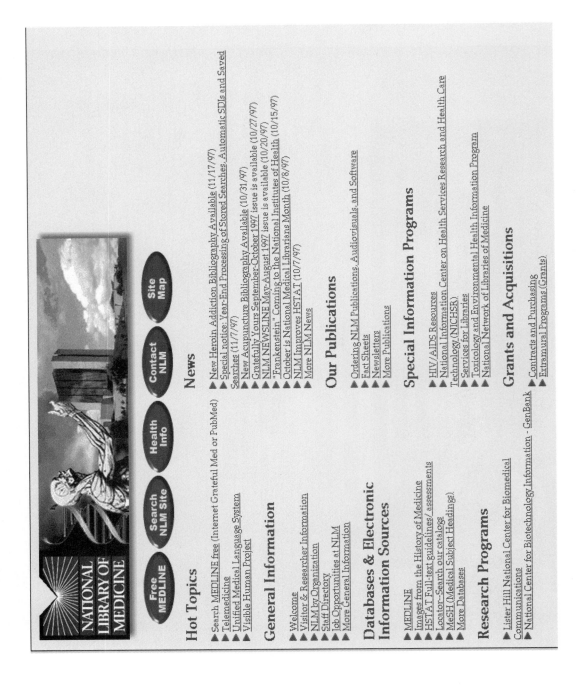

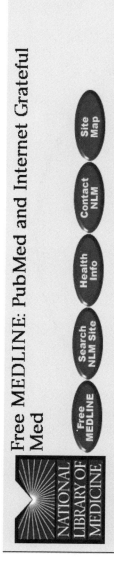

Free MEDLINE: PubMed and Internet Grateful Med

Free MEDLINE | **Search NLM Site** | **Health Info** | **Contact NLM** | **Site Map**

On June 26, 1997, NLM announced that its MEDLINE database of more than 8.8 million references to articles published in 3800 biomedical journals may be accessed free of charge on the World Wide Web. Two Web-based products, Internet Grateful Med and PubMed, provide this access. Below is a brief description of each system. For further information, see the documentation at each site. Health consumers are encouraged to discuss search results with their health care provider.

PubMed

- Provides free access to MEDLINE.
- Sets of related articles pre-computed for each article cited in MEDLINE
- Choice of Web search interfaces from simple keywords to advanced Boolean expressions. Field restrictions and MeSH index terms (main topics and subheadings) supported.
- Linkages to publishers' sites for full-text journals. Approximately 100 journals available, some by subscription only.
- Clinical query form with built-in search filters for diagnosis, therapy, and prognosis.
- Links to molecular biology databases of DNA/protein sequences and 3-D structure data.

Internet Grateful Med

- Provides free access to MEDLINE, AIDSLINE, HealthSTAR, AIDSDRUGS, AIDSTRIALS, DIRLINE, HISTLINE, HSRPROJ, OLDMEDLINE and SDILINE. A User ID Code is not needed.
- Can use Loansome Doc Document Delivery service (for domestic U.S. and Canadian health professional users; local charges may apply). A User ID Code is needed for this feature.
- Search features:
  - Utilize full range of Medical Subject Heading (MeSH) search features using UMLS Metathesaurus.
  - Ability to limit searches by language, publication type, age groups, etc., using pull-down menus.

U.S. National Library of Medicine (NLM)
http://www.nlm.nih.gov/
Last updated: 14 October 1997

PubMed

NLM's search service to access the 9 million citations in **MEDLINE** and Pre-MEDLINE (with links to participating on-line journals), and other related databases.

| Search | MEDLINE | for: |

Number of documents to display per page: 20

Pub. Date limit: No Limit

- Enter one or more search terms.
- Author names should be entered in the form Smith JB, but initials are optional.
- Journal titles may be entered in full, as valid MEDLINE abbreviations, or as ISSN numbers (see Journal Browser for more information).

Questions or comments? Write to the NCBI Help Desk.

NOTICE. The PubMed data are for personal use only. Users are responsible for complying with all copyright and licensing restrictions associated with data.

NATIONAL LIBRARY OF MEDICINE

Overview

Help

New/Noteworthy

Clinical Alerts

Advanced Search

Clinical Queries

Journal Browser

Internet Grateful Med

NLM Home

NCBI Home

NIH Home

Credits

Restrictions on use

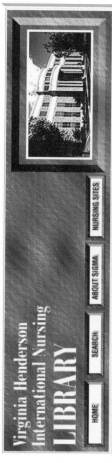

Virginia Henderson International Nursing
LIBRARY

HOME | SEARCH | ABOUT SIGMA | NURSING SITES

PROGRAMS | RESEARCH | MEMBERSHIP & CHAPTERS | PUBLICATIONS | PHILANTHROPY | LIBRARY

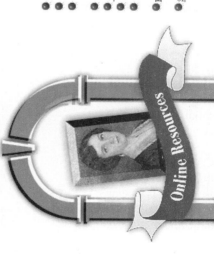

Online Resources

- Library News
- Frequently Asked Questions
- Questions / Suggestions

- Registry of Nursing Research
- The Online Journal of Knowledge Synthesis for Nursing
- Advanced Practice Nurses Conference
- Nursing Book Service

- Bibliographic Databases (CINAHLdirect(sm) ; MEDLINE®)

- Subscription Information

Search | Programs | Research | Membership & Chapters | Publications | Philanthropy | Library

Comments/Inquiries | Technical

Original: December 1996 Bruce L. Williams, Dale Bewley
Updated: 23 September 1997 Waiping Kam

URL: http://www.stti.iupui.edu/library/

Computerized Learning Resource
to Accompany
LoBiondo-Wood/Haber
NURSING RESEARCH:
Methods, Critical Appraisal, and Utilization

CD Installation Instructions

Windows 95

Insert the CD into your CD-ROM drive.
Click on the Start icon from the Taskbar. Select Run.
Type D:\nurseres (where D: is the drive designated for the CD-ROM) and press Enter.
The program will start automatically.

Windows 3.1

Insert the CD into your CD-ROM drive.
If Windows is not running, type WIN at the DOS prompt.
Select Run from the File menu.
Type D:\win31\nurseres (where D: is the drive designated for the CD-ROM) and press Enter.
The program will start automatically.

Macintosh

Insert the CD into your CD-ROM drive.
Double-click on the Nursing Research icon on the desktop.
Double-click on the Nursing Research icon in the folder.
The program will start automatically.

Technical Support

Technical support for this product is available at no charge by calling Mosbyís Technical Support Hotline between 9 a.m. and 6 p.m. CST, Monday through Friday. Inside the United States, call 1-800-692-9010. Outside the United States, call: 314-872-8370.

You may also contact Mosby Technical Support through e-mail: technical.support@mosby.com